SPRINGHOUSE NOTES

Pathophysiology

Kathy Lauer, RN, PhD
Assistant Professor
Rush University College of Nursing
Chicago

Sally A. Brozenec, RN, PhD
Assistant Professor
Rush University College of Nursing
Chicago

Springhouse Corporation
Springhouse, Pennsylvania

STAFF

Vice President
Matthew Cahill

Clinical Director
Judith Schilling McCann, RN, MSN

Editorial Director
Darlene Cooke

Art Director
John Hubbard

Managing Editor
David Moreau

Clinical Consultant
Beverly Ann Tscheschlog, RN

Clinical Editors
Clare Brabson, RN, BSN (clinical project manager); Jack Hogan, RN, CCRN, PHRN; Pamela Kovach, RN, BSN; Kate McGovern, RN, BSN, CCRN

Editors
Karen Diamond, Peter H. Johnson

Copy Editors
Brenna H. Mayer (manager), Gretchen Fee, Stacey A. Follin, Kathryn Marino, Pamela Wingrod

Designers
Arlene Putterman (associate art director), Mary Ludwicki

Manufacturing
Deborah Meiris (director), Patricia K. Dorshaw (manager), Otto Mezei (book production manager)

Editorial Assistants
Beverly Lane, Marcia Mills, Liz Schaeffer

A member of the Reed Elsevier plc group

Library of Congress Cataloging-in-Publication Data
Lauer, Kathy.
Pathophysiology / Kathy Lauer, Sally A. Brozenec.
      p.   cm. — (Springhouse notes)
    Includes bibliographical references and index.
    1. Physiology, Pathological—Outlines, syllabi, etc.
    2. Physiology, Pathological—Examinations, questions, etc.
    3. Nursing. I. Brozenec, Sally A. (Sally Ann), 1943- .
    II. Title. III. Series
    [DNLM: 1. Pathology outlines. 2. Pathology nurses'
    instruction. 3. Pathology examination questions. WY 18.2
    L372p 1999]
RB113.L325 1999
616.07—dc21.
DNLM/DLC   98-49667
ISBN 0-87434-964-8 (alk. paper)   CIP

Contents

Advisory Board, Contributors, and Reviewers

Jane V. McCloskey, RN, MSN
Faculty
Carolina College of Health Science
Charlotte, N. C.

Deborah B. Meehan, RN, MSN
Assistant Professor
College of Nursing and Health Pro-
  fessions
Marshall University
Huntington, W. Va.

Bonnie J. Nesbitt, RN, CS, PhD
Associate Professor
Viterbo College
LaCross, Wisc.

Wendy Woodward, RN, PhD
Professor and Chair
Department of Nursing
Humboldt State University
Arcata, Calif.

How to Use
Springhouse Notes

Springhouse Notes is a multivolume study guide series developed especially for nursing students. Each volume provides essential course material in outline format, enabling the student to review information efficiently.

Special features appear in every chapter to make information accessible and easy to remember. **Learning objectives** encourage the student to evaluate knowledge before and after study. **Chapter overview** highlights the chapter's major concepts. Within the outlined texts, key points are highlighted in color to facilitate a quick review of clinical information. Key points may include cardinal signs and symptoms, current theories, important steps in a nursing procedure, critical assessment findings, critical nursing interventions, or successful therapies and treatments. **Points to remember** summarize each chapter's major themes. **Study questions** then offer another opportunity to review material and assess knowledge gained before moving on to new information. **Critical thinking and application exercises** conclude each chapter, challenging students to expand on knowledge gained.

Other features appear throughout the book to facilitate learning: **Teaching tips** highlight key areas to address with patient teaching. **Clinical alerts** point out essential information on how to provide safe, effective care.

Pathophysiology **flowcharts** show disease progression in chart format. Difficult, frequently used, or sometimes misunderstood terms are indicated by SMALL CAPITAL LETTERS in the outline and defined in the glossary, appendix A; answers to the study questions appear in appendix B. Finally, a Windows-based software program (see diskette on inside back cover) poses 250 NCLEX-RN–style questions, formatted as required by the National Council of State Boards of Nursing, to assess your knowledge.

The Springhouse Notes volumes are designed as learning tools, not as primary information sources. When read conscientiously as a supplement to class attendance and textbook reading, Springhouse Notes can enhance understanding and help improve test scores and grades.

Cardiac Disorders

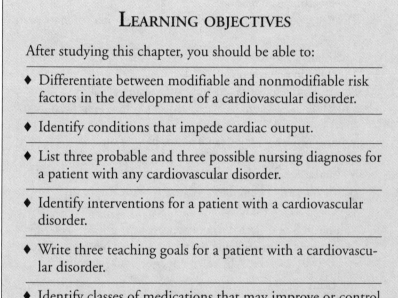

LEARNING OBJECTIVES

After studying this chapter, you should be able to:

♦ Differentiate between modifiable and nonmodifiable risk factors in the development of a cardiovascular disorder.

♦ Identify conditions that impede cardiac output.

♦ List three probable and three possible nursing diagnoses for a patient with any cardiovascular disorder.

♦ Identify interventions for a patient with a cardiovascular disorder.

♦ Write three teaching goals for a patient with a cardiovascular disorder.

♦ Identify classes of medications that may improve or control cardiac dysfunction.

CHAPTER OVERVIEW

The cardiovascular system begins its activity when the fetus is barely a month old and it's the last system to cease activity at the end of life.

The heart, arteries, veins, and lymphatics make up the cardiovascular system. These structures transport life-supporting oxygen and nutrients to CELLS, remove metabolic waste products, and carry hormones from one part of the body to another. Circulation requires normal heart function, which propels blood through the system by continuous rhythmic contractions.

Despite advances in disease detection and treatment, cardiovascular disease remains the leading cause of death in the United States. Heart attack, or myocardial infarction (MI), is the primary cause of cardiovascular-related deaths.

♦ I. Oxygen supply and demand

A. Critical balance — decrease in supply or increase in demand can threaten myocardial function
1. Major determinants of myocardial demand
   a. Heart rate
   b. Contractile force
   c. Muscle mass
   d. Ventricular wall tension
2. Tissue hypoxia most potent stimulus to increasing coronary perfusion

B. Valvular flow
1. Normally in one direction
2. Pressure gradient causes opening and closing of valves
3. Valve leaflets, or cusps, very responsive to even slight pressure differences
4. Valvular disease is major cause of low blood flow
   a. Allows regurgitation
   b. Increases cardiac workload
   c. May impede blood flow

C. CARDIAC OUTPUT (CO)
1. Volume of blood ejected from the heart per minute
2. Determined by multiplying the stroke volume (amount of blood ejected with each beat) by the number of beats per minute

D. Pump failure
1. Heart fails to meet tissues' metabolic requirements
2. Failure to perfuse may cause alteration in blood volume and vascular tone
3. Circulatory changes occur with changes in pressure
   a. Decreased pressure causes increased heart rate, increased force of contraction, vasoconstriction
   b. Increased pressure causes reflex slowing of heart rate, decreased force of contractions, vasodilation

♦ II. Risk factors

A. Controllable
1. Elevated serum lipid levels
2. Cigarette smoking
3. Sedentary lifestyle
4. Stress

5. Obesity

6. Excessive intake of saturated fats, carbohydrates, and salt

B. Uncontrollable

1. Age

2. Preexisting medical condition (diabetes mellitus, hypertension)

3. Family history

4. Male gender

5. Race

♦ III. Myocarditis

A. Pathophysiology

1. Focal or diffuse inflammation of the myocardium

2. Acute or chronic

3. Produces characteristic lesions (Aschoff bodies) in the interstitial tissue of the heart, which leads to formation of progressively fibrotic nodules and interstitial scars

4. Causes

   a. Viral infection (most common cause)

   b. Bacterial infection

   c. Hypersensitive immune reaction

   d. Radiation therapy

   e. Chemical poisons

   f. Parasitic infection

5. May induce myofibril degeneration that results in right- and left-sided heart failure

B. Assessment

1. Malaise

2. Fatigue

3. Dyspnea

4. Palpitations

5. Low-grade fever

6. Mild, continuous pressure or soreness in the chest

7. Recent febrile upper respiratory infection, viral pharyngitis, tonsillitis, or GI infection

8. Supraventricular and ventricular arrhythmias; heart block

9. Third and fourth heart sounds (S_3 and S_4); a faint first heart sound

C. Interventions

1. Bed rest

2. Monitor vital signs, hemodynamic variables

3. Antibiotics (as appropriate)

4. Low-sodium diet

5. Supplemental oxygen

◆ IV. Endocarditis

A. Pathophysiology
  1. Infection of the endocardium, heart valves, or cardiac prosthesis resulting from bacterial or fungal invasion
  2. Fibrin and platelets aggregate on the valve leaflets and engulf circulating bacteria or fungi, which flourish and produce friable verrucous vegetations
  3. Vegetations may embolize to the brain, spleen, kidneys, and lungs
  4. Vegetations may cause ulceration and necrosis or extend to the chordae tendineae, leading to their rupture and subsequent valvular insufficiency
  5. Classified as acute, subacute, or chronic
  6. Predisposing conditions
     a. I.V. drug abuse
     b. Valvular disease
     c. History of rheumatic or congenital heart defects
     d. Prosthetic heart valve

B. Assessment

  1. Intermittent fever, chills, or both, which may recur for weeks
  2. Loud, regurgitant murmur, typically of the underlying heart lesion
  3. Discovery of a new murmur in the presence of fever
  4. Embolization from vegetating lesions or diseased valvular tissue may produce typical features of splenic, renal, cerebral, or pulmonary infarction or of peripheral vascular occlusion
     a. Splenic: local pain, splenomegaly
     b. Renal: flank pain, hypertension, fever, nausea, vomiting
     c. Cerebral: headache, loss of consciousness or change in mental status, hemiparesis, aphasia
     d. Pulmonary: dyspnea, pleuritic chest pain, apnea, tachycardia
     e. Peripheral vascular occlusion: local pain, warmth, redness, edema
  5. Malaise
  6. Anorexia
  7. Dyspnea
  8. Tachycardia
  9. Splinter hemorrhages under fingernails and toenails

C. Interventions
  1. Bed rest
  2. Monitor vital signs and ECG rhythm
  3. Administer prescribed medications
     a. Antibiotics
     b. Analgesics
     c. Antipyretics
  4. Prosthetic or natural valve replacement

♦ V. Pericarditis

A. Pathophysiology
1. Inflammation of pericardium
   a. Acute: fibrous or effusive with serous, purulent, or hemorrhagic exudate
   b. Chronic (constrictive): dense and fibrous pericardial thickening, which causes a gradual increase in systemic venous pressure
2. Common causes
   a. Bacterial, fungal, or viral infection (infectious pericarditis)
   b. Neoplasms
   c. High-dose radiation to the chest
   d. Uremia, myxedema
   e. Hypersensitivity or autoimmune disease (systemic lupus erythematosus [SLE], rheumatoid arthritis)
   f. Drugs (such as hydralazine or procainamide)
   g. Idiopathic factors
   h. Postcardiac injury, MI, trauma, surgery
3. Incomplete healing may cause calcification and scarring, which may interfere with diastolic filling of ventricles, causing heart failure

**CLINICAL
ALERT**

B. Assessment
1. Sharp, sudden pain — usually over the sternum, which radiates to neck, shoulders, back, and arms
   a. Increases with deep inhalation
   b. Decreases when sitting up and leaning forward (pulls the heart away from the diaphragm and pleurae of the lungs)
2. Auscultation of pericardial friction rub (grating sound heard as the heart moves)
3. Gradual increase in systemic venous pressure, which produces signs and symptoms similar to those of right-sided heart failure
4. Signs of heart failure (dyspnea, orthopnea, and tachycardia) may indicate pericardial effusion (major complication of acute pericarditis)

C. Interventions
1. Bed rest (as long as fever and pain persist)
2. Administer prescribed medications
   a. Nonsteroidal anti-inflammatory drugs (NSAIDs)
   b. Corticosteroids (if NSAID is ineffective)
   c. Antibiotics
3. Surgical drainage: pericardiocentesis
4. Partial pericardectomy: if recurrent
5. Total pericardectomy: for constrictive pericarditis

♦ VI. Rheumatic fever and rheumatic heart disease

A. Pathophysiology

1. Systemic inflammatory disease of childhood that follows a group A beta-hemolytic streptococcal infection; often recurs and tends to run in families
2. Antibodies produced to combat streptococci react and produce characteristic lesions at specific tissue sites, mainly the heart, joints, central nervous system, skin, and subcutaneous tissues
3. Altered immune response probably is involved in its development or reoccurrence
4. In many cases leads to severe heart inflammation (carditis), which may affect the endocardium, myocardium, or pericardium during the acute phase; may result in valvular damage, especially to aortic and mitral valves

B. Assessment

1. Temperature of at least 100.4° F (38° C)
2. Positive for streptococcal infection that appeared a few days to 6 weeks earlier
3. Migratory joint pain (polyarthritis)
4. Swelling, redness, effusion of joints (mostly knees, ankles, elbows, and hips)
5. Nonpruritic, macular, transient rash (erythema marginatum) giving rise to red lesions with blanched centers
6. Fatigue; malaise
7. Limited range of motion
8. Subcutaneous nodules
   a. Firm, movable, nontender, approximately ⅛″ to ¾″ (3 to 20 mm) in diameter
   b. Usually near tendons or bony prominences of joints
9. Splenomegaly
10. Enlarged lymph nodes
11. Pericarditis
12. Chorea

C. Interventions

1. Administer prescribed medications
   a. Antibiotics: given during acute phase, then monthly to prevent recurrence (for 5 years or until age 21)
   b. Salicylates
   c. Corticosteroids
   d. Gold therapy
2. Bed rest initially (maybe up to 5 weeks), with progressive increase in physical activity
3. Check joints for swelling, pain, redness, reduced mobility

4. Surgery
   a. Valve surgery
   b. Commissurotomy, valvuloplasty, or replacement
   c. Joint replacement or synovectomy

♦ VII. Valvular disorders

A. Pathophysiology
   1. Three types of mechanical disruption
      a. STENOSIS: narrowing of the valve opening
      b. Incomplete closure of the valve: regurgitation, insufficiency, or incompetence
      c. Prolapse of the valve
   2. May lead to heart failure
   3. Causes
      a. Endocarditis (most common)
      b. Congenital defect
      c. Inflammation
      d. Trauma
      e. Degenerative changes

B. Assessment and diagnostic tests (see *Types of valvular heart disease,* pages 8 to 10, for information on assessment and diagnostic tests)

C. Interventions
   1. Depend on nature and severity of associated symptoms
   2. Monitor vital signs, intake and output, and hemodynamic variables
   3. Diet: low-sodium
   4. Administer oxygen and medications as prescribed
      a. Digoxin
      b. Diuretics
      c. Anticoagulants
      d. Prophylactic antibiotics before and after surgery and dental care
   5. Valvuloplasty
   6. Valve replacement

♦ VIII. Coronary artery disease (CAD)

A. Pathophysiology
   1. Narrowing or obstruction of the coronary arteries that impedes blood flow and causes angina pectoris (classic symptom)
   2. CAD has several causes
      a. Atherosclerosis: an accumulation of fatty, fibrous plaques that narrow the lumen of the coronary arteries
      b. Vasospasm: spontaneous, sustained contraction of one or more coronary arteries
      c. Embolus: a clot, or thrombus that traveled to a coronary artery

(Text continues on page 10.)

Types of valvular heart disease

CAUSES AND INCIDENCE	CLINICAL FEATURES
Aortic insufficiency • Results from rheumatic fever, syphilis, hypertension, endocarditis, or may be idiopathic • Associated with Marfan syndrome • Most common in males • Associated with ventricular septal defect, even after surgical closure	• Dyspnea, cough, fatigue, palpitations, angina, syncope • Pulmonary venous congestion, heart failure, pulmonary edema (left-sided heart failure), "pulsating" nail beds (Quincke's sign) • Rapidly rising and collapsing pulses (biferious pulse), cardiac arrhythmias, wide pulse pressure in severe insufficiency • Auscultation reveals a third heart sound (S_3) and a diastolic blowing murmur at left sternal border. • Palpation and visualization of apical impulse in chronic disease
Aortic stenosis • Results from congenital aortic bicuspid valve (associated with coarctation of the aorta), congenital stenosis of valve cusps, rheumatic fever, or atherosclerosis in the elderly • Most common in males	• Exertional dyspnea, paroxysmal nocturnal dyspnea, fatigue, syncope, angina, palpitations • Pulmonary venous congestion, heart failure, pulmonary edema • Diminished carotid pulses, decreased cardiac output (CO), cardiac arrhythmias; may have alternating pulse • Auscultation reveals systolic murmur at base or in carotids and, possibly, a fourth heart sound.
Mitral insufficiency • Results from rheumatic fever, hypertrophic cardiomyopathy, mitral valve prolapse syndrome, myocardial infarction, severe left-sided heart failure, or ruptured chordae tendineae • Associated with other congenital anomalies, such as transposition of the great arteries • Rare in children without other congenital anomalies	• Orthopnea, dyspnea, fatigue, angina, palpitations • Peripheral edema, jugular vein distention, hepatomegaly (right-sided heart failure)
Mitral stenosis • Results from rheumatic fever (most common cause) • Most common in females • May be associated with other congenital anomalies	• Tachycardia, crackles, pulmonary edema • Auscultation reveals a holosystolic murmur at apex, a possible split second heart sound (S_2) and an S_3

Types of valvular heart disease (continued)

CAUSES AND INCIDENCE	CLINICAL FEATURES
Mitral valve prolapse syndrome • Cause unknown. Researchers speculate that metabolic or neuroendocrine factors cause constellation of signs and symptoms • Most commonly affects young women but may occur in both sexes and in all age-groups	• Dyspnea on exertion, paroxysmal nocturnal dyspnea, orthopnea, weakness, fatigue, palpitations • Peripheral edema, jugular vein distention, ascites, hepatomegaly (right-sided heart failure in severe pulmonary hypertension) • Crackles, cardiac arrhythmias (atrial fibrillation), signs and symptoms of systemic emboli • Auscultation reveals a loud first heart sound or opening snap and a diastolic murmur at the apex.
Pulmonic insufficiency • May be congenital or may result from pulmonary hypertension • May rarely result from prolonged use of pressure monitoring catheter in the pulmonary artery	• May produce no signs or symptoms • Chest pain, palpitations, headache, fatigue, exercise intolerance, dyspnea, light-headedness, syncope, mood swings, anxiety, panic attacks • Auscultation typically reveals a mobile, midsystolic click, with or without a mid- to late-systolic murmur.
Pulmonic stenosis • Results from congenital stenosis of valve cusp or rheumatic heart disease (uncommon) • Associated with other congenital heart defects such as tetralogy of Fallot	• Dyspnea, weakness, fatigue, chest pain • Peripheral edema, jugular vein distention, hepatomegaly (right-sided heart failure) • Auscultation reveals diastolic murmur in pulmonic area.
Tricuspid insufficiency • Results from right-sided heart failure, rheumatic fever and, rarely, trauma and endocarditis • Associated with congenital disorders	• Asymptomatic or symptomatic with exertional dyspnea, fatigue, chest pain, syncope • May lead to peripheral edema, jugular vein distention, hepatomegaly (right-sided heart failure) • Auscultation reveals a systolic murmur at the left sternal border, a split S_2 with a delayed or absent pulmonic component.

(continued)

Types of valvular heart disease (continued)

CAUSES AND INCIDENCE	CLINICAL FEATURES
Tricuspid stenosis • Results from rheumatic fever • May be congenital • Associated with mitral or aortic valve disease • Most common in women	• Dyspnea and fatigue • May lead to peripheral edema, jugular vein distention, hepatomegaly, and ascites (right-sided heart failure) • Auscultation reveals possible S_3 and systolic murmur at lower left sternal border that increases with inspiration. • May be symptomatic with dyspnea, fatigue, syncope • Possibly peripheral edema, jugular vein distention, hepatomegaly, and ascites (right-sided heart failure) • Auscultation reveals diastolic murmur at lower left sternal border that increases upon inhalation.

3. Obstructed blood vessels decrease perfusion and reduce myocardial oxygen supply; when oxygen demand exceeds what the diseased vessel can supply, localized myocardial ischemia results
   a. Transient ischemia causes reversible changes at the cellular and tissue levels, depressing myocardial function, and may lead to tissue injury or necrosis
   b. Oxygen deprivation forces the myocardium to shift from aerobic to anaerobic metabolism, causing lactic acid to accumulate, which reduces cellular pH (acidosis)
4. Impaired left ventricular function results from combination of hypoxia, reduced energy availability, and acidosis
   a. Reduced stroke volume lowers CO
   b. Left-sided heart pressure and pulmonary artery wedge pressure (PAWP) increase
5. Predisposing factors include:
   a. Age: greater risk over 40 years
   b. Sex: males have greater incidence
   c. Race: more prevalent in whites
   d. Positive family history
   e. Hypertension
   f. Increased low-density lipoproteins (LDLs) and very low-density lipoproteins (VLDLs) and decreased high-density lipoproteins (HDLs)
   g. Smoking

      h. Stress or type-A personality

      i. Obesity

      j. Excessive intake of saturated fats, carbohydrates, or salt

      k. Inactivity

      l. Diabetes mellitus

B. Assessment findings

  1. Hypertension

  2. Angina (four major forms); a burning, squeezing, or tightness in the substernal or precordial chest that may radiate to the left arm, neck, jaw, or shoulder

    a. Stable

      (1) Pain is predictable in frequency and duration and can be relieved with nitrates and rest

      (2) Usually associated with activity

    b. Unstable

      (1) Pain increases in frequency and duration and is more easily induced

      (2) May occur at rest

    c. Prinzmetal's or variant: due to unpredictable coronary artery spasm

    d. Microvascular: impairment of vasodilator reserve causes angina-like chest pain in a patient with normal coronary arteries

CLINICAL ALERT

  3. Myocardial infarction: severe and prolonged anginal pain generally suggests MI, with potential fatal arrhythmias and mechanical failure

  4. Heart failure

C. Interventions

  1. Assess cardiovascular status

  2. Administer oxygen and medications as prescribed

    a. Antihyperlipidemic agents

    b. Nitrates

    c. Beta-adrenergic blockers

    d. Calcium channel blockers

    e. Analgesics

    f. Antianxiety agents

  3. Monitor vital signs, intake and output, hemodynamic variables, ECG, and laboratory studies

  4. Diet control

    a. Low-calorie, low-sodium, low-cholesterol, low-fat diet

    b. Increased dietary fiber

  5. Lifestyle modification

  6. Thrombolytic therapy

  7. Intra-aortic balloon pump (IABP)

  8. Percutaneous transluminal coronary angioplasty (PTCA)

  9. Laser angioplasty

TEACHING TIPS
Patient with coronary artery disease

Be sure to include the following topics in your teaching plan for the patient with coronary artery disease:
1. Reduce serum lipid levels by following a low-fat, low-cholesterol diet.
2. Exercise daily.
3. Stop smoking.
4. Reduce weight.
5. Reduce or prevent high blood pressure.

10. Atherectomy
11. Provide information about the American Heart Association
12. For additional teaching tips, see *Patient with coronary artery disease*

◆ IX. Myocardial infarction

A. Pathophysiology
  1. Narrowing and eventual obstruction of the coronary arteries from plaque accumulation, embolus, or vasospasm
    a. Occlusion of the circumflex coronary artery causes antero-lateral wall infarction
    b. Occlusion of the proximal left anterior descending (LAD) coronary artery causes anterior wall infarction
    c. Occlusion of the LAD artery causes anteroseptal wall infarction
    d. Occlusion of the anterior right coronary artery (RCA) or one of its branches causes inferior wall infarction
    e. Occlusion of proximal RCA causes right ventricular infarction
    f. Occlusion of circumflex branch of left coronary artery causes posterior wall infarction.
    g. Right ventricular infarctions can also accompany inferior wall infarctions and may cause right-sided heart failure.
  2. Death of myocardial cells from inadequate perfusion and oxygenation has several effects
    a. Reduced contractility with abnormal wall function
    b. Altered left ventricular compliance
    c. Reduced stroke volume
    d. Reduced ejection fraction
    e. Elevated left ventricular end-diastolic pressure
  3. Scar tissue that forms in the necrotic area inhibits contractility
    a. Compensatory mechanisms (vascular constriction, increased heart rate, renal retention of sodium and water) attempt to maintain CO
    b. Heart failure or cardiogenic shock may develop

4. In transmural (Q-wave) MI, tissue damage extends through all my-ocardial layers; in subendocardial (non-Q-wave) MI, usually only the innermost layer is damaged

5. Predisposing factors
   a. Age
   b. Diabetes mellitus
   c. Hypertension
   d. Excessive intake of saturated fats, carbohydrates, or salt
   e. Obesity
   f. Family history of CAD
   g. Sedentary lifestyle
   h. Stress
   i. Use of amphetamines or cocaine
   j. Smoking

B. Assessment
   1. Crushing substernal pain
      a. May radiate to the jaw, back, and arms
      b. Can be described as heavy, squeezing, or crushing
      c. Lasts longer than anginal pain
      d. Is unrelieved by rest or nitroglycerin
      e. May not be present (asymptomatic or silent MI), especially in diabetic and elderly patients
   2. Dyspnea
   3. Nausea and vomiting
   4. Anxiety, restlessness
   5. Diaphoresis
   6. Pallor
   7. Arrhythmias
   8. Low-grade fever
   9. Fatigue and weakness
   10. Hypotension or hypertension

C. Interventions
   1. Obtain an ECG reading during acute pain; serial ECGs
   2. Monitor vital signs, intake and output, hemodynamic variables, laboratory studies, and ECG results
   3. Administer oxygen and medications as prescribed
      a. Nitrates
      b. Antiarrhythmics
      c. Anticoagulants; antiplatelet agents
      d. Antihypertensives
      e. Angiotensin-converting enzyme inhibitors
      f. Beta-adrenergic blockers
      g. Calcium channel blockers
      h. Thrombolytic therapy

TEACHING TIPS
Patient with myocardial infarction

Be sure to include the following topics in your teaching plan for the patient with myocardial infarction:
1. Monitor activities of daily living; avoid activities that induce fatigue or chest pain.
2. Complete a cardiac rehabilitation program.
3. Avoid crowds or individuals with infections.
4. Reduce weight.
5. Stop smoking.
6. Control or prevent hypertension.
7. Follow the prescribed medication regimen.

4. Diet: low-calorie, low-cholesterol, low-fat (for additional teaching tips, see *Patient with myocardial infarction*)
5. IAPB
6. PTCA
7. Laser angioplasty
8. Vascular stents
9. Atherectomy
10. Transmyocardial laser revascularization
11. Coronary artery bypass graft
12. Cardiac rehabilitation

◆ X. Heart failure

A. Pathophysiology
1. Caused by impairment of heart's pumping ability; results in inability to adequately perfuse body tissues
2. Muscle contractility is usually reduced and CO declines while venous input to the ventricle remains the same
3. Muscular compensatory mechanisms
   a. Short-term adaptation: Frank-Starling curve; ventricular muscle dilates and increases force of contraction
   b. Long-term adaptation: ventricular hypertrophy increases the heart muscle's ability to contract and eject its volume of blood into circulation
4. Neuroendocrine compensatory mechanisms
   a. Increased sympathetic activity and increased catecholamines result in increased blood pressure, systemic vascular resistance and heart rate, with shunting of blood to vital organs
   b. Renin-angiotensin-aldosterone system activation leads to increased sodium and water retention

5. Right-sided heart failure
   a. Caused by ineffective right ventricular contractility or filling
   b. May be caused by profound backward flow due to left-sided heart failure, acute right ventricular infarct, pulmonary embolus, chronic pulmonary disease or hypertension, tricuspid or pulmonic valve disease
   c. May lead to decreased CO and systemic edema
6. Left-sided heart failure
   a. Caused by ineffective left ventricular contractility or filling
   b. May be caused by left ventricular infarct, systemic hypertension, aortic or mitral valve disease, myocarditis, and cardiomyopathy
   c. May lead to pulmonary congestion or edema, decreased CO, and right-sided heart failure
7. Forward heart failure
   a. Caused by inadequate delivery of blood to the systemic or pulmonic arterial system
   b. Direct result of increased afterload
8. Backward heart failure
   a. Ventricles fail to empty
   b. Results in progressive accumulation of fluid in pulmonic or systemic circulation or both
9. Acute heart failure
   a. Rapid onset of signs and symptoms leaves no time for compensatory mechanisms to respond
   b. Fluid status is usually normal or low; sodium and water retention doesn't occur
10. Chronic heart failure
    a. Signs and symptoms have been present for a period of time
    b. Compensatory mechanisms have taken place
    c. Fluid volume overload persists
    d. Structural changes occur, such as dilation or hypertrophy
11. Low-output failure
    a. Failure to maintain systemic CO adequate to perfuse tissues
    b. Types
       (1) Systolic: contractility problem
       (2) Diastolic: filling problem
12. High-output failure
    a. Failure of an abnormally high CO to meet an increased demand for increased blood flow
    b. Results from pregnancy, thyrotoxicosis, anemia, fever, valvular insufficiency
13. Predisposing factors
    a. See right- and left-sided failure, low- and high-output failure (points A. 5, A. 6, A. 11, and A. 12 above)
    b. Noncompliance with treatment regimen for cardiac disease

B. Assessment
1. Fatigue, malaise, weakness
2. Exertional and paroxysmal nocturnal dyspnea, tachypnea
3. Neck vein engorgement, hepatojugular reflux
4. Marked hepatomegaly, splenomegaly
5. Tachycardia
6. Palpitations
7. Dependent pitting edema
8. Unexplained, steady weight gain
9. Nausea; anorexia, abdominal fullness, ascites
10. Chest tightness
11. Slowed mental response; restlessness
12. Hypotension; narrow pulse pressure
13. Gallop rhythms S_3 and S_4; inspiratory crackles on auscultation; cough, cyanosis
14. Diaphoresis

C. Interventions
1. Goal is to control or treat precipitating factors
2. Administer oxygen and medications as prescribed
   a. Diuretics
   b. Inotropics
   c. Sympathomimetics
   d. Vasodilators
   e. Nitrates
   f. Analgesics (morphine)
   g. Antianxiety agents
3. Monitor vital signs, intake and output, hemodynamic variables, ECG
4. Bed rest; high Fowler's position
5. Antiembolism stockings
6. IABP
7. Daily weights

◆ XI. Dilated cardiomyopathy

A. Pathophysiology
1. Also called congestive cardiomyopathy
2. Primary disease of the myocardium, causes gross dilation of all four heart chambers and gives the heart a globular shape
3. Thrombi commonly develop in the dilated chambers due to blood pooling and STASIS, which may lead to embolization
4. Usually affects middle-aged men, but can occur in any group
5. Possible causes
   a. Infectious agents, such as myocarditis

   b. Metabolic agents that cause endocrine and electrolyte disorders
      and nutritional deficiencies
   c. Muscle disorders
   d. Infiltrative disorders
   e. Sarcoidosis
   f. Rheumatic fever
   g. Alcoholism
   h. Use of doxorubicin, cyclophosphamide, cocaine, and fluorouracil
   i. Autosomal dominant or recessive or X-linked inheritance pat-
      terns
   j. Pregnancy
 6. Insidious onset; may lead to end-stage refractory heart failure

B. Assessment
 1. Difficulty breathing; orthopnea, exertional dyspnea, paroxysmal
    nocturnal dyspnea, bibasilar crackles
 2. Fatigue
 3. Dry cough at night
 4. Palpitations
 5. Vague chest pain
 6. Narrow pulse pressure
 7. Irregular rhythms
 8. S_3 and S_4 gallop rhythms
 9. Pansystolic murmur
 10. Ascites
 11. Peripheral edema
 12. JVD

C. Interventions
 1. Correct underlying cause; discontinue alcohol
 2. Monitor vital signs, intake and output, hemodynamic variables,
    ECG
 3. Bedrest
 4. Administer oxygen and medications as prescribed
    a. Digitalis glycosides
    b. Diuretics
    c. Anticoagulants
    d. Vasodilators
    e. Antiarrhythmics
    f. Corticosteroids
 5. Low-sodium diet with supplemental vitamins
 6. Heart transplantation
 7. Avoid myocardial depressants, including alcohol.
 8. Intracardiac ventricular defibrillation (ICVD)

◆ XII Hypertrophic cardiomyopathy (HCM)

A. Pathophysiology

1. Also known as idiopathic hypertrophic subaortic stenosis, hypertropic obstructive cardiomyopathy, muscular aortic stenosis, or asymmetric septal hypertrophy
2. Primary disease of the cardiac muscle characterized by left ventricular, right ventricular, or biventricular hypertrophy and an unusual cellular hypertrophy of the upper ventricular septum
3. Changes in the heart result in a pressure difference that leads to an obstruction of blood outflow from the left ventricle
4. Hypertrophy of the intraventricular septum causes altered function of the anterior leaflet of the mitral valve and mitral regurgitation
5. Myocardial wall may stiffen over time, causing increased resistance to blood entering the right atrium and an increase in diastolic filling pressures
6. CO may be low, normal, or high, depending on whether the stenosis is obstructive or nonobstructive
7. In 50% of cases, HCM is transmitted genetically as an autosomal dominant trait. Other causes are unknown

B. Assessment

1. Atrial fibrillation (most common arrhythmia), supraventricular and ventricular arrhythmias
2. Orthopnea
3. Exertional dyspnea
4. Syncope
5. Fatigue
6. Edema
7. Tachypnea
8. Migratory joint pain
9. Abdominal pain
10. Chest pain

C. Interventions

1. Monitor vital signs, intake and output, hemodynamic variables, ECG
2. Administer prescribed medications
   a. Beta-adrenergic blockers
   b. Calcium channel blockers
   c. Heparin (during atrial fibrillation)
   d. Antiarrythmics
   e. Avoid vasodilators, sympathetic stimulators, and inotropics, because they worsen the obstruction
3. Ventricular myotomy with or without myectomy
4. Mitral valve replacement

**CLINICAL
ALERT**

5. Dual chamber pacemaker
6. ICVD

◆ XIII. Restrictive cardiomyopathy

A. Pathophysiology
1. A disorder of cardiac muscle marked by restricted ventricular filling (due to left ventricular hypertrophy) and endocardial fibrosis and thickening, resulting in low CO
2. Idiopathic or result of myocardial infiltrations such as amyloidosis (infiltration of amyloid into the intracellular spaces in the myocardium, endocardium, and subendocardium)
3. Diabetes, endomyocardial fibrosis, postradiation

B. Assessment
1. Fatigue, weakness
2. Dyspnea, orthopnea, paroxysmal nocturnal dyspnea
3. Chest pain
4. Peripheral edema
5. Liver engorgement with ascites
6. Peripheral cyanosis
7. Pallor
8. S_3 and S_4 gallop rhythms
9. Systolic murmurs of mitral and tricuspid insufficiency
10. Arrhythmias
11. JVD

C. Interventions
1. Monitor vital signs, intake and output, and hemodynamic variables, ECG
2. Administer oxygen and medications as prescribed
   a. Digitalis glycosides
   b. Diuretics
   c. Vasodilators
   d. Anticoagulants
   e. Antiarrythmics
   f. Steroids
3. Diet: low-sodium

◆ XIV. Hypovolemic shock

A. Pathophysiology
1. Reduced intravascular blood volume causes circulatory dysfunction and inadequate tissue perfusion
2. Due to low blood flow and decreased oxygen, cellular metabolism shifts from aerobic to anaerobic pathways, resulting in an accumulation of lactic acid and leading to metabolic (lactic) acidosis

What happens in hypovolemic shock

In hypovolemic shock, vascular fluid volume loss causes extreme tissue hypoperfusion. Internal fluid losses can result from hemorrhage or third space fluid shifting. External fluid loss can result from severe bleeding or from severe diarrhea, diuresis, or vomiting. Inadequate vascular volume leads to decreased venous return and cardiac output. The resulting drop in arterial blood pressure activates the body's compensatory mechanisms in an attempt to increase vascular volume. If compensation is unsuccessful, decompensation and death may occur.

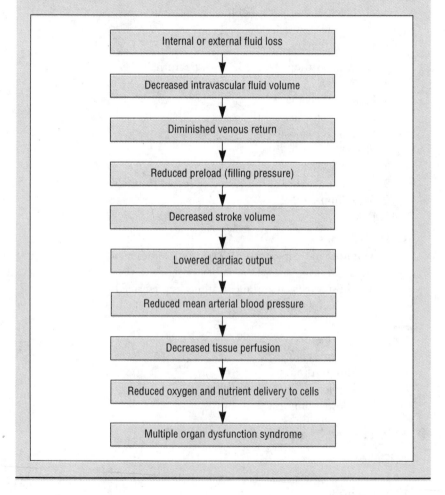

3. May lead to irreversible cerebral and renal damage, cardiac arrest, and ultimately death (see *What happens in hypovolemic shock*)
4. Usually results from acute blood loss (one-fifth of total volume)
   a. GI bleeding

b. Internal hemorrhage (hemothorax)

c. External hemorrhage (accidental or surgical trauma)

d. Any condition that reduces circulating intravascular plasma volume or other body fluids (severe burns, diarrhea, vomiting, dehydration, third spacing)

B. Assessment

1. Hypotension with narrowing pulse pressure
2. Decreased sensorium
3. Tachycardia
4. Rapid, shallow respirations, cyanosis
5. Reduced urine output (< 20 ml/hour)
6. Cold, clammy skin
7. Restlessness, anxiety
8. Increased capillary refill time

C. Interventions

1. Prompt and adequate blood, blood component, and fluid replacement
2. Identification of bleeding site or other avenue of fluid loss
3. Control of bleeding by direct measures (application of pressure and elevation of extremity)
4. Monitor vital signs, intake and output, and laboratory values
5. Surgery to correct bleeding site or other avenue of fluid loss
6. Administer oxygen and medications as prescribed
   a. Steroids
   b. Vasopressors
   c. Analgesics
   d. Diuretics
7. CVP or pulmonary capillary wedge pressure monitoring

◆ XV. Cardiogenic shock

A. Pathophysiology

1. Failure of heart muscle to pump adequately, resulting in diminished CO that severely impairs tissue perfusion; also called pump failure
2. Reflects severe left-sided heart failure
3. Compensatory mechanisms
   a. Aortic and carotid baroreceptors initiate sympathetic nervous responses
   b. Heart rate, left ventricular filling pressures, and resistance to flow increase to enhance venous return to heart
   c. Initially stabilizes patient but later causes deterioration with rising demands of compromised myocardium
4. Shock may result from
   a. MI (most common cause): 15% of those whose area of infarction exceeds 40% of the muscle mass

   b. Myocardial ischemia

   c. Papillary muscle dysfunction

   d. End-stage CAD or cardiomyopathy

   e. Severe arrhythmias

B. Assessment

  1. Cold, clammy skin

  2. Decreased blood pressure, narrowing pulse pressure

  3. Tachycardia

  4. Rapid, shallow respirations; cyanosis

  5. Oliguria (< 20 ml/hour)

  6. Decreased sensorium; restlessness; anxiety

  7. Gallop rhythm with faint heart sounds

  8. Increased capillary refill time

C. Interventions

  1. Monitor vital signs, intake and output, hemodynamic variables, laboratory values, and ECG

  2. Administer oxygen and medications as prescribed

   a. Vasopressors

   b. Inotropics

   c. Vasodilators

   d. Antianxiety agents

  3. IABP

  4. Left ventricular assist device

◆ XVI. Ventricular aneurysm

A. Pathophysiology

  1. Outpouching (almost always of the left ventricle) that produces ventricular wall dysfunction in 10% to 20% of patients with MI

  2. Necrosis reduces the ventricular wall to a thin fibrous sheath, which stretches and forms a separate noncontractile sac due to intracardiac pressure

  3. Noncontractile sac causes AKINESIA, DYSKINESIA, ASYNERGIA, and asynchrony, which causes the remaining normally functioning myocardial fibers to increase the force of contraction to maintain stroke volume and CO

  4. A portion of stroke volume is lost to passive distention of the noncontractile sac

  5. Aneurysm enlarges but seldom ruptures

B. Assessment

  1. Arrhythmias

  2. Palpitations

  3. Weakness on exertion

  4. Fatigue

  5. Angina

6. Visible or palpable systolic precordial bulge

C. Interventions
1. Routine physical assessments, periodic electrocardiography to follow condition
2. Monitor vital signs, ECG rhythm
3. Administer prescribed antiarrhythmic medication
4. Cardioversion
5. Aneurysmectomy with myocardial revascularization

◆ XVII. Cardiac tamponade

A. Pathophysiology
1. Rapid rise in intrapericardial pressure, usually from blood or fluid accumulation in the pericardial sac, that impairs diastolic filling of the heart
2. Reduced blood flow into the ventricles decreases the amount of blood that can be pumped out of the heart with each contraction; more fluid accumulates in the pericardial sac, further limiting the amount of blood that can fill the chamber during the next cardiac cycle
3. Causative factors
   a. Effusion, such as in cancer, bacterial infections, tuberculosis and, rarely, rheumatic fever
   b. Hemorrhage caused by trauma, such as penetrating wound to the chest or surgery, or invasive procedure, such as central venous catheterization
   c. Hemorrhage from nontraumatic causes, such as rupture of the heart or great vessels and anticoagulant therapy in a patient with pericarditis
   d. Viral, postradiation, or idiopathic pericarditis
   e. Acute MI
   f. Chronic renal failure during dialysis
   g. Drug reaction from procainamide, hydralazine, minoxidil, isoniazid, penicillin, methysergide, or daunorubicin
   h. Connective tissue disorders, such as rheumatoid arthritis, SLE, rheumatic fever, vasculitis, and scleroderma
4. Dressler's syndrome (no known cause)
5. Amount of fluid needed to cause tamponade: 200 ml (rapid filling) to 2,000 ml (slow accumulation as pericardial sac adapts to increase)

CLINICAL ALERT
B. Assessment
1. Classic features: Beck's triad
   a. Elevated CVP with neck vein distention
   b. Muffled heart sounds
   c. Paradoxical pulse (inspiratory drop in systolic blood pressure greater than 15 mm Hg)

2. Orthopnea
3. Diaphoresis
4. Anxiety
5. Restlessness
6. Cyanosis
7. Weak, rapid peripheral pulse

  C. Interventions
1. Removal of accumulated blood or fluid:
   a. Pericardiocentesis
   b. Surgical creation of an opening (pericardial window)
   c. Insertion of a drain into the pericardial sac
2. Monitor vital signs, hemodynamics, and ECG
3. Volume loading (for hypotension) with I.V. normal saline solution and albumin
4. Administer prescribed medications, such as inotropics
5. Blood transfusion (in traumatic injury)
6. Heparin antagonist such as protamine sulfate (in heparin-induced tamponade)
7. Vitamin K (in warfarin-induced tamponade)
8. Resection of pericardium

◆ XVIII. Cardiac arrhythmias

  A. Pathophysiology
1. Abnormal electrical conduction or automaticity that changes heart rate and rhythm
2. Generally classified according to origin (ventricular or supraventricular)
3. Vary in severity from mild, asymptomatic, and requiring no treatment to life-threatening and requiring immediate resuscitation

  B. Interventions (see *Types of cardiac arrhythmias*)

(Text continues on page 32.)

Types of cardiac arrhythmias

This chart reviews many common cardiac arrhythmias and outlines their features, causes, and treatments. Use a normal electrocardiogram strip, if available, to compare normal cardiac rhythm configurations with the rhythm strips below. Characteristics of normal rhythm include:
- ventricular and atrial rates of 60 to 100 beats/minute
- regular and uniform QRS complexes and P waves
- PR interval of 0.12 to 0.20 second
- QRS duration <0.12 second
- identical atrial and ventricular rates, with constant PR interval.

ARRHYTHMIA AND FEATURES	CAUSES	TREATMENT
Sinus arrhythmia • Irregular lengthening and shortening of R-R intervals • Normal P wave preceding each QRS complex	• A normal variation of normal sinus rhythm in athletes, children, and elderly people • Also seen in digitalis toxicity and inferior wall myocardial infarction (MI)	• Follow advanced cardiac life support (ACLS) guidelines for bradycardia if rate drops below 40 beats/minute and patient is symptomatic (for example, has hypotension)
Sinus tachycardia • Atrial and ventricular rates regular • Rate >100 beats/minute; rarely, >160 beats/minute • Normal P wave preceding each QRS complex	• Normal physiologic response to fever, exercise, anxiety, pain, dehydration; may also accompany shock, left-sided heart failure, cardiac tamponade, hyperthyroidism, anemia, hypovolemia, pulmonary embolism, anterior wall MI • May also occur with atropine, epinephrine, isoproterenol, quinidine, caffeine, alcohol, and nicotine use	• Correction of underlying cause
Sinus bradycardia • Regular atrial and ventricular rates • Rate <60 beats/minute • Normal P wave preceding each QRS complex	• Normal in well-conditioned heart, as in an athlete • Increased intracranial pressure; increased vagal tone due to straining during defecation, vomiting, intubation, mechanical ventilation; sick sinus syndrome; hypothyroidism; inferior wall MI • May also occur with anticholinesterase, beta blocker, digoxin, and morphine use	• For low CO, dizziness, weakness, altered level of consciousness, or low blood pressure: follow ACLS protocol for administration of atropine • Temporary pacemaker or isoproterenol if atropine fails; may need permanent pacemaker

(continued)

Types of cardiac arrhythmias (continued)

ARRHYTHMIA AND FEATURES	CAUSES	TREATMENT
Sinoatrial (SA) arrest or block (sinus arrest) • Atrial and ventricular rhythms normal except for missing complex • Normal P wave preceding each QRS complex • Pause not equal to a multiple of the previous R-R interval	• Acute infection • Coronary artery disease (CAD), degenerative heart disease, acute inferior wall MI • Vagal stimulation, Valsalva's maneuver, carotid sinus massage • Digitalis, quinidine, or salicylate toxicity • Pesticide poisoning • Pharyngeal irritation caused by endotracheal (ET) intubation • Sick sinus syndrome	• Treat signs and symptoms with I.V. atropine • Temporary or permanent pacemaker for repeated episodes
Wandering atrial pacemaker • Atrial and ventricular rates vary slightly • Irregular PR interval • P waves irregular with changing configuration, indicating that they're not all from SA node or single atrial focus; may appear after the QRS complex • QRS complexes uniform in shape but irregular in rhythm	• Rheumatic carditis due to inflammation involving the SA node • Digitalis toxicity • Sick sinus syndrome	• No treatment if patient is asymptomatic • Treatment of underlying cause if patient is symptomatic
Premature atrial contraction (PAC) • Premature, abnormal-looking P waves that differ in configuration from normal P waves • QRS complexes after P waves, except in very early or blocked PACs • P wave may be buried in the preceding T wave or identified in the preceding T wave	• Coronary or valvular heart disease, atrial ischemia, coronary atherosclerosis, heart failure, acute respiratory failure, chronic obstructive pulmonary disease (COPD), electrolyte imbalance, and hypoxia • Digitalis toxicity; use of aminophylline, adrenergics, or caffeine • Anxiety	• If PACs increase in frequency (in presence of acute MI or other acute myocardial problem), digoxin, quinidine, verapamil, or propranolol; after revascularization surgery, propranolol • Treatment of underlying cause

Types of cardiac arrhythmias (continued)

ARRHYTHMIA AND FEATURES	CAUSES	TREATMENT
Paroxysmal atrial tachycardia (paroxysmal supraventricular tachycardia) 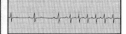 • Atrial and ventricular rates regular • Heart rate >160 beats/minute; rarely exceeds 250 beats/minute • P waves regular but aberrant; difficult to differentiate from preceding T wave • P wave preceding each QRS complex • Sudden onset and termination of arrhythmia • Tends to be recurrent	• Intrinsic abnormality of AV conduction system • Physical or psychological stress, hypoxia, hypokalemia, cardiomyopathy, congenital heart disease, MI, valvular disease, Wolff-Parkinson-White syndrome, cor pulmonale, hyperthyroidism, systemic hypertension • Digitalis toxicity; use of caffeine, marijuana, or central nervous system stimulants	• If patient is unstable, prepare for immediate cardioversion. • If patient is stable, prepare for vagal stimulation, Valsalva's maneuver, carotid sinus massage. • Adenosine by rapid I.V. bolus injection to rapidly convert arrhythmia • If patient is stable, determine QRS complex width. For wide complex width, follow ACLS protocol for lidocaine and procainamide. For narrow complex width and normal or elevated blood pressure, follow ACLS protocol for verapamil and consider digoxin, beta blockers, and diltiazem. For narrow complex width with low or unstable blood pressure (and for ineffective drug response for others), use synchronized cardioversion.
Atrial flutter 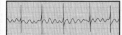 • Atrial rhythm regular rate; 250 to 450 beats/minute • Ventricular rate variable, depending on degree of atrioventricular (AV) block (usually 60 to 100 beats/minute) • Sawtooth P-wave configuration possible (F waves) • QRS complexes uniform in shape, but generally irregular in rate	• Heart failure, tricuspid or mitral valve disease, pulmonary embolism, cor pulmonale, inferior wall MI, carditis • Digitalis toxicity	• If patient is unstable with a ventricular rate >150 beats/minute, prepare for immediate cardioversion. • If patient is stable, drug therapy may include diltiazem, beta blockers, verapamil, digoxin, procainamide, or quinidine.

(continued)

Types of cardiac arrhythmias *(continued)*

ARRHYTHMIA AND FEATURES	CAUSES	TREATMENT
Atrial fibrillation • Atrial rhythm grossly irregular; rate >400 beats/minute • Ventricular rate grossly irregular • QRS complexes of uniform configuration and duration • PR interval indiscernible • No P waves, or P waves that appear as erratic, irregular, baseline fibrillatory waves	• Heart failure, COPD, thyrotoxicosis, constrictive pericarditis, ischemic heart disease, sepsis, pulmonary embolus, rheumatic heart disease, hypertension, mitral stenosis, atrial irritation, complication of coronary bypass or valve replacement surgery	• If patient is unstable with a ventricular rate >150 beats/minute, prepare for immediate cardioversion. • If patient is stable, drug therapy may include diltiazem, beta blockers, verapamil, digoxin, procainamide, quinidine, amiodarone, and ibutilide. • In some patients with refractory atrial fibrillation uncontrolled by drugs, radiofrequency catheter-induced ablation may be required.
Junctional rhythm • Atrial and ventricular rates regular • Atrial rate 40 to 60 beats/minute • Ventricular rate usually 40 to 60 beats/minute (60 to 100 beats/minute is accelerated junctional rhythm) • P waves preceding, hidden within (absent), or after QRS complex; usually inverted if visible • PR interval (when present) <0.12 second • QRS complex configuration and duration normal, except in aberrant conduction	• Inferior wall MI or ischemia, hypoxia, vagal stimulation, sick sinus syndrome • Acute rheumatic fever • Valve surgery • Digitalis toxicity	• Atropine for symptomatic slow rate • Pacemaker insertion if patient is refractory to drugs • Discontinuation of digoxin, if appropriate

Types of cardiac arrhythmias (continued)

ARRHYTHMIA AND FEATURES	CAUSES	TREATMENT
Junctional contractions (junctional premature beats) • Atrial and ventricular rhythms irregular • P waves inverted; may precede, be hidden within, or follow QRS complex • PR interval < 0.12 second if P wave precedes QRS complex • QRS complex configuration and duration normal	• MI or ischemia • Digitalis toxicity and excessive caffeine or amphetamine use	• Correction of underlying cause • Atropine, as ordered • Discontinuation of digoxin if appropriate • May require pacemaker
First-degree AV block • Atrial and ventricular rhythms regular • PR interval > 0.20 second • P wave preceding each QRS complex • QRS complex normal	• May be seen in a healthy person • Inferior wall myocardial ischemia or infarction, hypothyroidism, hypokalemia, hyperkalemia • Digitalis toxicity; use of quinidine, procainamide, or propranolol	• Cautious use of digoxin • Correction of underlying cause • Possibly atropine if PR interval exceeds 0.26 second or bradycardia develops
Second-degree AV block (Mobitz I or Wenckebach) • Atrial rhythm regular • Ventricular rhythm irregular • Atrial rate exceeds ventricular rate • PR interval progressively, but only slightly, longer with each cycle until QRS complex disappears (dropped beat); PR interval shorter after dropped beat	• Inferior wall MI, cardiac surgery, acute rheumatic fever, and vagal stimulation • Digitalis toxicity; use of propranolol, quinidine, or procainamide	• Treatment of underlying cause • Atropine or temporary pacemaker for symptomatic bradycardia • Discontinuation of digoxin, if appropriate

(continued)

Types of cardiac arrhythmias (continued)

ARRHYTHMIA AND FEATURES	CAUSES	TREATMENT
Second-degree AV block (Mobitz II) • Atrial rate regular • Ventricular rhythm regular or irregular, with varying degree of block • PR interval constant • P-P interval constant • QRS complexes periodically absent	• Severe CAD, anterior wall MI, acute myocarditis • Digitalis toxicity	• Atropine or Isoproterenol for symptomatic bradycardia (follow ACLS guidelines) • Temporary or permanent pacemaker • Discontinuation of digoxin, if appropriate
Third-degree AV block (complete heart block) • Atrial rate regular • Ventricular rate slow and regular • No relation between P waves and QRS complexes • No constant PR interval • QRS interval normal (nodal pacemaker) or wide and bizarre (ventricular pacemaker)	• Inferior or anterior wall MI, congenital abnormality, rheumatic fever, hypoxia, postoperative complication of mitral valve replacement, Lev's disease (fibrosis and calcification that spreads from cardiac structures to the conductive tissue), Lenègre's disease (conductive tissue fibrosis) • Digitalis toxicity	• Atropine or isoproterenol for symptomatic bradycardia (follow ACLS guidelines) • Temporary or permanent pacemaker
Junctional tachycardia • Atrial rate >100 beats/minute; however, P wave may be absent, hidden in QRS complex, or preceding T wave • Ventricular rate >100 beats/minute • P wave may be present or absent; inverted in lead II • QRS complex normal • Onset of rhythm sudden, occurring in bursts	• Myocarditis, cardiomyopathy, inferior wall MI or ischemia, acute rheumatic fever, complication of valve replacement surgery • Digitalis toxicity	• Temporary atrial pacemaker to override the rhythm • Carotid sinus massage, elective cardioversion • Follow ACLS guidelines for narrow complex tachycardia • Discontinuation of digoxin, if appropriate

Types of cardiac arrhythmias (continued)

ARRHYTHMIA AND FEATURES	CAUSES	TREATMENT
Premature ventricular contraction (PVC) 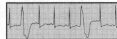 • Atrial rate regular • Ventricular rate irregular • QRS complex premature, usually followed by a complete compensatory pause • QRS complex wide and distorted, usually >0.14 second • Premature QRS complexes occurring singly, in pairs, or in threes; alternating with normal beats; focus from one or more sites • Ominous when clustered, multifocal, with R wave on T pattern	• Heart failure; old or acute myocardial ischemia, infarction, or contusion; myocardial irritation by ventricular catheter, such as a pacemaker; hypercapnia; hypokalemia, hypocalcemia • Drug toxicity (digitalis glycosides, aminophylline, tricyclic antidepressants, beta-adrenergics [isoproterenol or dopamine]) • Caffeine, tobacco, or alcohol use • Psychological stress, anxiety, pain, exercise	• If warranted, I.V. lidocaine, I.V. procainamide, or I.V. bretylium • Treatment of underlying cause • Discontinuation of drug causing toxicity • I.V. potassium chloride if PVC induced by hypokalemia
Ventricular tachycardia 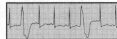 • Ventricular rate 140 to 220 beats/minute, regular or irregular • QRS complexes wide, bizarre, and independent of P waves • P waves not discernible • May start and stop suddenly	• Myocardial ischemia, infarction, or aneurysm; CAD; rheumatic heart disease; mitral prolapse; heart failure; cardiomyopathy; ventricular catheters; hypokalemia; hypercalcemia; pulmonary embolism • Digitalis glycoside, procainamide, epinephrine, or quinidine toxicity • Anxiety	• With pulse: If hemodynamically stable with ventricular rate <150 beats/minute, follow ACLS protocol for administration of lidocaine, procainamide, or bretylium; if drugs are ineffective, initiate synchronized cardioversion. • If ventricular rate >150 beats/minute, follow ACLS protocol for immediate synchronized cardioversion, followed by antiarrhythmic agents. • Pulseless: initiate cardiopulmonary resuscitation (CPR); follow ACLS protocol for defibrillation, endotracheal (ET) intubation, and administration of epinephrine, lidocaine, bretylium, magnesium sulfate, or procainamide.

(continued)

Types of cardiac arrhythmias (continued)

ARRHYTHMIA AND FEATURES	CAUSES	TREATMENT
Ventricular fibrillation • Ventricular rhythm rapid and chaotic • QRS complexes wide and irregular; no visible P waves	• Myocardial ischemia or infarction, R-on-T phenomenon, untreated ventricular tachycardia, hypokalemia, hyperkalemia, hypercalcemia, alkalosis, electric shock, hypothermia • Digitalis, epinephrine, or quinidine toxicity	• Pulseless: Initiate CPR; follow ACLS protocol for defibrillation, ET intubation, and administration of epinephrine, lidocaine, bretylium, magnesium sulfate, or procainamide.
Asystole • No atrial or ventricular rate or rhythm • No discernible P waves, QRS complexes, or T waves	• Myocardial ischemia or infarction, aortic valve disease, heart failure, hypoxemia, hypokalemia, severe acidosis, electric shock, ventricular arrhythmias, AV block, pulmonary embolism, heart rupture, cardiac tamponade, hyperkalemia, electromechanical dissociation • Cocaine overdose	• Continue CPR; follow ACLS protocol for ET intubation, administration of epinephrine, and atropine, and possible transcutaneous pacing.

POINTS TO REMEMBER

◆ The focus of nursing management in cardiovascular disorders is to increase blood supply — and thus oxygenation — to tissues.

◆ Alterations in CO affect every system in the body.

◆ The impact of cardiovascular disease can be reduced by altering modifiable risk factors.

◆ Complaints of chest pain or cardiac symptoms or both have increased significance in a patient with peripheral vascular disorders.

◆ A unilateral finding in the assessment of peripheral circulation has greater significance than bilateral findings.

STUDY QUESTIONS

To evaluate your understanding of this chapter, answer the following questions in the space provided; then compare your responses with the correct answers in appendix B, page 289.

1. What are the signs and symptoms of right- and left-sided heart failure?_____

   _____

2. What are four causes of hypovolemic shock? _____

   _____

3. How does Beck's triad relate to cardiac tamponade?_____

   _____

4. What is the major pathophysiologic effect of cardiac tamponade? _____

   _____

5. What are the assessment findings in the patient with acute pulmonary edema? _____

CRITICAL THINKING AND APPLICATION EXERCISES

1. Observe a cardiac catheterization. Prepare an oral presentation for your fellow students describing the procedure.

2. Develop a chart describing the major drug classes used for treating angina.

3. Obtain a 3-day food history from a fellow student. Evaluate the information for possible cardiac risk factors and identify ways to modify them.

4. Follow a patient with a cardiac disorder from admission to discharge. Develop a patient-specific plan of care.

Vascular Disorders

CHAPTER OVERVIEW

Interruption of blood flow through vessels causes tissue damage and, eventually, death. Quick assessment of decreased blood flow needs rapid intervention to resume adequate HOMEOSTASIS. Nursing care needs to focus on evaluation of circulation and promotion of optimal blood flow.

♦ **I. Circulation**

    A. Vessels

        1. Arteries: adjust to the volume of blood leaving the heart

        2. Veins: return blood to the heart

        3. Capillaries

            a. Thin-walled

            b. Pass blood to the veins

    c. Site of movement of oxygen, carbon dioxide, and nutrients at tissue level

B. Blood flow changes

    1. Aneurysms develop slowly; weakened vessel wall

    2. Occlusion: blockage in flow

    3. Narrowed vessels caused by lesions, thrombus, spasm of vessel

    4. Increased viscosity (from dehydration or other causes)

    5. Valvular diseases causing turbulent blood flow

◆ II. Risk factors

A. Controllable

    1. Elevated serum lipid levels

    2. Hypertension

    3 Cigarette smoking

    4. Diabetes mellitus

    5. Sedentary lifestyle

    6. Trauma

    7. Obesity

    8. Excessive intake of saturated fats, carbohydrates, and salt

B. Uncontrollable

    1. Age

    2. Male gender

    3. Family history

    4. Race

◆ III. Aneurysms

A. Pathophysiology

    1. Abnormal localized dilation in the vessel wall, usually an artery

    2. Classification

        a. Saccular (berry): unilateral pouchlike bulge with a narrow neck

        b. Fusiform: spindle-shaped bulge encompassing entire vessel diameter

        c. Dissecting: hemorrhagic separation of medial layer of artery, creating a false lumen

        d. False: pulsating hematoma resulting from trauma

    3. Locations

        a. Thoracic aortic: ascending aorta (most common), transverse or descending part of the aorta

        b. Abdominal: occurs in aorta between the renal arteries and iliac branches

        c. Femoral and popliteal: femoral and popliteal arteries, generally affecting both legs

        d. Cerebral: circle of Willis, especially anterior circulation

 4. Causes
   a. Atherosclerosis
   b. Hypertension
   c. Trauma
   d. Fungal infection
   e. Congenital defects
   f. Syphilis
   g. Degenerative changes

B. Assessment
   1. Thoracic aortic aneurysm
      a. Ascending
         (1) Severe pain that extends to neck, shoulders, back, and abdomen
         (2) Bradycardia
         (3) Aortic insufficiency
         (4) Difference in blood pressure between right and left arms
      b. Descending
         (1) Sharp, sudden pain, usually between shoulder blades
         (2) Aortic insufficiency without murmur
         (3) Blood pressure remains the same in both arms
      c. Transverse
         (1) Sharp, sudden pain, radiating to shoulders
         (2) Hoarseness, dyspnea, dysphagia, dry cough
   2. Abdominal aneurysm
      a. Pulsating mass in periumbilical area
      b. Systolic BRUIT over aorta
      c. Tenderness on palpation; lumbar pain that radiates to flank and groin (signifies enlargement)
   3. Femoral and popliteal aneurysms
      a. Pain in popliteal space
      b. Edema and venous distention
      c. ISCHEMIA in leg or foot
      d. Palpation of pulsating mass above or below inguinal ligament

**CLINICAL
ALERT**

▮

   4. Cerebral aneurysm
      a. Sudden and severe headache
      b. Nuchal rigidity
      c. Photophobia
      d. Loss of consciousness
      e. Increased intracranial pressure
      f. Nausea, vomiting
      g. Focal neurologic defects
      h. Cranial nerve defects

C. Interventions
   1. Monitor vital signs, intake and output, and laboratory values

2. Administer oxygen and medications as prescribed
   a. Analgesics
   b. Antibiotics
   c. Antihypertensives
   d. Negative inotropics
   e. Calcium channel blockers
   f. Vasopressors
3. Fluids
4. Resection of aneurysm with graft replacement or aneurysmal clipping
5. Embolization, balloon dilation

◆ IV. Thrombophlebitis

A. Pathophysiology
1. Acute condition characterized by inflammation and thrombus formation, which initiates a chemical inflammatory process in the vessel epithelium, leading to fibrosis
2. Deep vein thrombosis
   a. Intramuscular or intermuscular
   b. Affects small veins or large veins, usually of lower extremities
   c. Progressive, may lead to pulmonary EMBOLISM
   d. Results from endothelial damage and accelerated blood clotting and reduced blood flow
   e. Predisposing factors: prolonged bed rest, trauma, surgery, childbirth, use of oral contraceptives
3. Superficial vein thrombophlebitis
   a. Subcutaneous
   b. Self-limiting; seldom leads to pulmonary embolism
   c. Results from trauma, infection, I.V. drug abuse, chemical irritation due to extensive use of I.V. route for medication and diagnostic tests

B. Assessment
1. Clinical signs and symptoms vary with the site and length of affected vein
2. Deep vein thrombosis
   a. Severe pain at site
   b. Fever, chills
   c. Malaise
   d. Swelling and cyanosis of affected limb
3. Superficial thrombophlebitis
   a. Heat at site
   b. Pain, tenderness
   c. Swelling
   d. Induration

C. Interventions
1. Bed rest with elevation of the affected extremity
2. Warm, moist soaks
3. Administer prescribed medications
    a. Analgesics
    b. Anticoagulants
    c. Anti-inflammatory agents
    d. Thrombolytic agents
4. Antiembolism stockings
5. Embolectomy
6. Insertion of umbrella filter

◆ V. Raynaud's disease

A. Pathophysiology
1. Arterioplastic disorder
2. Episodic severe vasospasm in the small peripheral arteries and arterioles, precipitated by exposure to cold or psychological stress
3. Occurs bilaterally; usually affects the hands or, less often, the feet
4. Possible causes
    a. Intrinsic vascular wall hyperreactivity to cold
    b. Increased vasomotor tone due to sympathetic stimulation
    c. Antigen-antibody immune response

B. Assessment
1. Cyanosis of fingers or toes after exposure to cold or psychological stress
2. Numbness and tingling of digits
3. Relief of signs and symptoms with warmth

C. Interventions
1. Avoidance of cold, mechanical, or chemical injury and psychological stress
2. Cessation of smoking
3. Avoidance of vasoconstrictors, especially caffeine and over-the-counter medications such as Neo-Synephrine (phenylephrine HCl); for additional teaching tips, see *Patient with Raynaud's disease*
4. Sympathectomy if ischemic ulcers occur (< 25% of patients)
5. Biofeedback
6. Vasodilators
7. Calcium channel blockers

◆ VI. Buerger's disease

A. Pathophysiology
1. Inflammatory, nonartheromatous occlusive condition

TEACHING TIPS
Patient with Raynaud's disease

Be sure to include the following topics in your teaching plan for the patient with Raynaud's disease:
1. Avoid precipitating factors
2. Consider use of heat packets or battery-operated heated gloves.
3. Quit or limit smoking.
4. Avoid vasoconstrictive substances such as caffeine. Check all over-the-counter medications for vasoconstrictive components.
5. Use relaxation exercises to decrease stress.

2. Causes segmental lesions and subsequent thrombus formation in the small and medium arteries (and sometimes the veins), resulting in decreased blood flow to feet and legs
3. May produce ulceration and, eventually, gangrene
4. Cause is unknown; however, possible hypersensitivity to nicotine may contribute

B. Assessment
1. INTERMITTENT CLAUDICATION of the instep and digits, aggravated by exercise and relieved by rest
2. Exposure to cold causes cyanosis and numbness; later, redness, warmth and tingling
3. Impaired peripheral pulses
4. Migratory superficial thrombophlebitis
5. Local hair loss

C. Interventions
1. Exercise program that uses gravity to fill and drain the blood vessels
2. Smoking cessation (for additional teaching tips, see *Patient with Buerger's disease,* page 40)
3. Lumbar sympathectomy: increases blood supply to the skin (severe cases)
4. Amputation: for nonhealing ulcers, intractable pain, or gangrene

◆ VII. Arterial occlusive disease

A. Pathophysiology
1. Obstruction or narrowing of the lumen of the aorta and its major branches
2. Interrupts blood flow to the legs and feet; may affect the carotid, vertebral, innominate, subclavian, mesenteric, and celiac arteries
3. Causes severe ischemia, skin ulceration, and gangrene

TEACHING TIPS
Patient with Buerger's disease

Be sure to include the following topics in your teaching plan for the patient with Buerger's disease:
1. Quit or limit smoking.
2. If taking vasodilating medications for this disorder, avoid effects of orthostatic hypotension:
a. Do not stand up too quickly from a sitting or lying down position.
b. If feeling lightheaded or dizzy, sit or lie down. Report frequent episodes to the doctor.
3. Perform Buerger-Allen exercises:
a. Lie down with legs elevated 45 to 90 degrees for 2 to 3 minutes.
b. Sit up with feet dependent for 5 to 10 minutes.
c. Flex, extend, pronate and supinate, each foot three times.
d. Lie flat for 10 minutes.

    4. Predisposing factors
       a. Atherosclerosis
       b. Smoking
       c. Aging
       d. Family history of vascular disorders
       e. Myocardial infarction
       f. Cerebrovascular accident

B. Assessment
    1. Pain distal to the location of occlusion
    2. Absence of pulse
    3. Signs and symptoms dependent on severity and location of occlusion (see *Types of arterial occlusive disease*)

C. Interventions
    1. Elimination of smoking
    2. Hypertension control
    3. Embolectomy
    4. Thromboendarterectomy
    5. Patch grafting
    6. Bypass
    7. Thrombolytic therapy
    8. Atherectomy
    9. Balloon or laser angioplasty
   10. Stents

Types of arterial occlusive disease

SITE OF OCCLUSION	SIGNS AND SYMPTOMS
Carotid arterial system • Internal carotids • External carotids	Neurologic dysfunction: transient ischemic attacks (TIAs) due to reduced cerebral circulation produce unilateral sensory or motor dysfunction (transient monocular blindness, hemiparesis), possible aphasia or dysarthria, confusion, decreased mentation, and headache. These recurrent clinical features usually last 5 to 10 minutes, but they may persist up to 24 hours and may herald a stroke. Absent or decreased pulsation with an auscultatory bruit over the affected vessels.
Vertebrobasilar system • Vertebral arteries • Basilar arteries	Neurologic dysfunction: TIAs of brain stem and cerebellum produce binocular visual disturbances, vertigo, dysarthria, and "drop attacks" (falling down without loss of consciousness). Less common than carotid TIA.
Innominate • Brachiocephalic artery	Neurologic dysfunction: signs and symptoms of vertebrobasilar occlusion. Indications of ischemia (claudication) of right arm; possible bruit over right side of neck.
Subclavian artery	Subclavian steal syndrome (characterized by the backflow of blood from the brain through the vertebral artery on the same side as the occlusion, into the subclavian artery distal to the occlusion); clinical effects of vertebrobasilar occlusion and exercise-induced arm claudication. Possible gangrene, usually limited to the digits.
Mesenteric artery • Superior (most commonly affected) • Celiac axis • Inferior	Bowel ischemia, infarct necrosis, and gangrene; sudden, acute abdominal pain; nausea and vomiting; diarrhea; leukocytosis; and shock due to massive intraluminal fluid and plasma loss.
Aortic bifurcation (saddle-block occlusion, a medical emergency associated with cardiac embolization)	Sensory and motor deficits (muscle weakness, numbness, paresthesia, paralysis), and signs and symptoms of ischemia (sudden pain; cold, pale legs with decreased or absent peripheral pulses) in both legs.
Iliac artery (Leriche's syndrome)	Intermittent claudication of lower back, buttocks, and thighs, relieved by rest; absent or reduced femoral or distal pulses; possible bruit over femoral arteries; impotence in males.
Femoral and popliteal arteries (associated with aneurysm formation)	Intermittent claudication of the calves on exertion; ischemic pain in feet; pretrophic pain (heralds necrosis and ulceration); leg pallor and coolness; blanching of feet on elevation; gangrene; no palpable pulses in ankles and feet.

◆ VIII. Hypertension

A. Pathophysiology

1. An intermittent or sustained elevation of systolic blood pressure of 140 mm Hg or higher or a diastolic pressure of 90 mm Hg or higher

2. Causes

   a. Changes in the arteriolar bed cause increased resistance

   b. Abnormally increased tone of vasomotor systems causes increased peripheral vascular resistance

   c. Increase in blood volume caused by conditions of renal or hormonal dysfunction

   d. Increase in arteriolar thickening caused by genetic factors, leading to increased peripheral vascular resistance

   e. Abnormal renin release resulting in the formation of angiotensin II, which constricts the arterioles and increases blood volume

3. Essential (primary or idiopathic) hypertension

   a. Most common

   b. Insidious onset

   c. Initially benign; may progress to a malignant state

4. Secondary hypertension

   a. Related to underlying disease, which raises peripheral vascular resistance or CO

   b. Chronic renal disease is most common cause

   c. Other causes include renal parenchymatous disease, pheochromocytoma, primary aldosteronism, Cushing's syndrome, diabetes mellitus, pregnancy, coarctation of the aorta, neurologic disease, or dysfunction of the thyroid, pituitary, or parathyroid gland

5. Malignant hypertension

   a. Severe, fulminant

   b. May arise from essential or secondary hypertension

6. Signs and symptoms of hypertension result from vascular changes in the heart, brain, eye, or kidney due to damage to the intima of small vessels, resulting in fibrin accumulation and possible clotting

   a. Heart: MI, heart failure

   b. Retina: blindness

   c. Brain: cerebral vascular accident

   d. Kidneys: chronic renal failure

7. Risk factors

   a. Family history

   b. Race (most common in African-Americans)

   c. Stress

   d. High intake of saturated fats, sodium, or alcohol

   e. Obesity

   f. Tobacco use

   g. Sedentary lifestyle

TEACHING TIPS
Patient with hypertension

Be sure to include the following topics in your teaching plan for the patient with hypertension:
1. Set up a plan for lifestyle changes to reduce weight.
2. Stop smoking.
3. Reduce dietary intake of salt.
4. Consume no more than 2 ounces of hard liquor, 8 ounces of wine, or 24 ounces of beer per day.
5. Know your hypertensive medications and potential interactions with other drugs or food.

    h. Aging
    i. Oral contraceptives
B. Assessment
  1. Elevated blood pressure
    a. Stage 1 (mild): 140 to 159/90 to 99 mm Hg
    b. Stage 2 (moderate): 160 to 179/100 to 109 mm Hg
    c. Stage 3 (severe): 180 to 209/110 to 119 mm Hg
    d. Stage 4 (very severe, typically symptomatic): 210/120 mm Hg
  2. Headache
  3. Signs and symptoms of target organ disease:
    a. Visual disturbances or visual loss
    b. Left ventricular hypertrophy
    c. Proteinuria, edema, azotemia
    d. Dizziness
    e. Papilledema
    f. Heart failure: dependent edema, pulmonary edema, jugular venous distention (JVD), splenomegaly, hepatomegaly
    g. Cerebral ischemia: motor or sensory changes, visual disturbances, dysphasia, cranial nerve abnormalities
C. Interventions
  1. Lifestyle modification
  2. Diet modification: low-sodium, low-calorie, low-cholesterol, low-fat; restrict alcohol and caffeine
  3. Administer prescribed medications
    a. Diuretics
    b. Vasodilators
    c. Calcium channel blockers
    d. Beta-adrenergic or alpha-adrenergic blockers
    e. Angiotensin-converting enzyme inhibitors
  4. Monitor vital signs, intake and output, laboratory values

5. Provide information about the American Heart Association

6. For additional teaching tips, see *Patient with hypertension,* page 43

POINTS TO REMEMBER

◆ A unilateral finding in the assessment of peripheral circulation has greater significance than bilateral findings.

◆ The focus of nursing management in vascular disorders is to obtain rapid treatment and promote adequate circulation.

◆ The impact of vascular disease can be reduced by the alteration of modifiable risk factors.

STUDY QUESTIONS

To evaluate your understanding of this chapter, answer the following questions in the space provided; then compare your responses with the correct answers in appendix B, page 289.

1. What are the four classifications of aneurysms? _____

_____

2. What is the most common aneurysm site?_____

_____

3. What are three predisposing factors for the development of deep vein thrombosis?_____

_____

CRITICAL THINKING AND APPLICATION EXERCISES

1. Observe an arteriogram. Prepare an oral report describing the evaluation of blood flow through vessels.

2. Develop a chart depicting the different classifications of aneurysms.

3. Follow a patient with a vascular disorder. Identify risk factors and develop a plan of care that may improve the outcome of the patient's illness.

Respiratory Disorders

LEARNING OBJECTIVES

After studying this chapter, you should be able to:

♦ Differentiate between modifiable and nonmodifiable risk factors in the development of a respiratory disorder.

♦ List three nursing interventions for a patient with a respiratory disorder.

♦ Write three goals for teaching a patient with a respiratory disorder.

♦ Understand the function of respiratory passages and lungs.

♦ Know the types of treatments specific for respiratory disorders.

CHAPTER OVERVIEW

Working with the cardiovascular system, the respiratory system ensures that the tissues receive sufficient oxygen and that carbon monoxide is removed promptly. To maintain homeostasis, it must perform this gas exchange under widely varying external conditions and internal demands.

Every body cell needs oxygen. Without it, death would occur within minutes. Therefore, the health care professional must be familiar with the respiratory system and be prepared to maintain it as needed. A thorough assessment is essential to planning and implementing appropriate patient care. The assessment includes a complete history, physical examination, diagnostic testing, identification of modifiable and nonmodifiable risk factors, and information related to the psychosocial impact of respiratory dysfunction on the patient.

◆ I. Conducting airways

A. Upper airway
  1. Structures
     a. Nose
     b. Mouth
     c. Pharynx
     d. Larynx
  2. Function
     a. Allows air flow into and out of lungs
     b. Warms, humidifies, and filters inspired air
     c. Protects the lower airway from foreign matter
  3. Obstruction
     a. Caused by trauma, tumors, mucus, foreign objects, inflammation
     b. Leads to hypoxemia; progresses to hypoxia, loss of consciousness, and death

B. Lower airway
  1. Structures
     a. Trachea
     b. Right and left main stem bronchi
     c. Five secondary bronchi
     d. Bronchioles: contain alveolar ducts and ALVEOLI
  2. Function
     a. Facilitate gas exchange
     b. Clearance mechanism: cough reflex, mucociliary
     c. Immunologic responses
     d. Pulmonary injury response
  3. Obstruction
     a. Caused by inflammation, tumors, foreign bodies, trauma
     b. Leads to respiratory distress and death

◆ II. Gas exchange

A. Ratio of ventilation to perfusion ($\dot{V}/\dot{Q}$ ratio); see *Understanding ventilation and perfusion*

B. Breathing mechanics: affected by adult respiratory distress syndrome (ARDS), thoracic deformity, muscle spasm, abdominal distention, and drugs
  1. Lung volume and capacity
  2. Compliance: changes may occur in the lung or chest wall

Understanding ventilation and perfusion

Effective gas exchange depends on the relationship between ventilation and perfusion, or the $\dot{V}/\dot{Q}$ ratio. The diagrams below show what happens when the $\dot{V}/\dot{Q}$ ratio is normal and abnormal.

Normal ventilation and perfusion

When ventilation and perfusion are matched, unoxygenated blood from the venous system returns to the right ventricle through the pulmonary artery to the lungs, carrying carbon dioxide. The arteries branch into the alveolar capillaries. Gas exchange takes place in the alveolar capillaries.

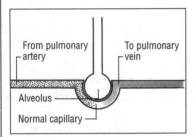

Inadequate perfusion (dead-space ventilation)

When the $\dot{V}/\dot{Q}$ ratio is high, as shown below, ventilation is normal, but alveolar perfusion is reduced or absent. Note the narrowed capillary, indicating poor perfusion. This commonly results from a perfusion defect, such as pulmonary embolism or a disorder that decreases cardiac output.

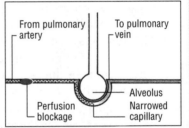

Inadequate ventilation (shunt)

When the $\dot{V}/\dot{Q}$ ratio is low, pulmonary circulation is adequate but not enough oxygen is available to the alveoli for normal diffusion. A portion of the blood flowing through the pulmonary vessels does not become oxygenated.

Inadequate ventilation and perfusion (silent unit)

The silent unit indicates an absence of ventilation and perfusion to the lung area. The silent unit might help compensate for a $\dot{V}/\dot{Q}$ imbalance by delivering blood flow to better-ventilated lung areas.

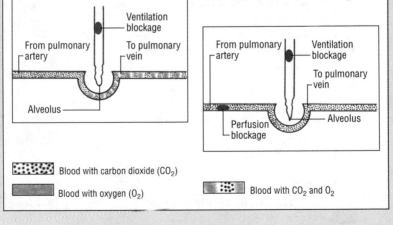

3. Resistance to air flow may occur in lung tissue, chest wall, or airways

C. Neurochemical control
   1. Respiratory center
      a. Located in the lateral medulla oblongata of the brain stem
      b. Consists of neurons that determine the rate and depth of respiration
   2. Chemoreceptors
      a. Respond to hydrogen ion concentration of arterial blood, the partial pressure of arterial carbon dioxide ($Paco_2$), and the partial pressure of arterial oxygen (Pao_2)
      b. Respond indirectly to arterial blood by sensing changes in the pH of cerebrospinal fluid

◆ III. Adult respiratory distress syndrome

A. Pathophysiology
   1. Form of noncardiac pulmonary edema that can quickly lead to acute respiratory failure
   2. Also known as shock, stiff, wet, white, or DaNang lung; may follow a direct or indirect injury to pulmonary microcirculation
   3. Characterized by diffuse injury to alveolocapillary membrane and decreased surfactant production
   4. Fluid accumulates in the lung interstitium, alveolar spaces, and small airways, causing the lung to stiffen, which impairs ventilation and reduces oxygenation of pulmonary capillary blood
   5. Hypoxemia and respiratory acidosis develop, causing an increased drive for ventilation, leading to metabolic acidosis (lactic acidosis)
   6. Causes
      a. Trauma (most common cause)
      b. Anaphylaxis
      c. Aspiration of gastric contents
      d. Diffuse pneumonia
      e. Drug overdose, toxin exposure
      f. Near-drowning
      g. Oxygen toxicity
      h. Coronary artery bypass grafting
      i. Hemodialysis
      j. Leukemia, tuberculosis, pancreatitis
      k. Venous air embolism
      l. Diabetes mellitus, uremia
      m. Sepsis
      n. Shock
      o. Disseminated intravascular coagulation
      p. Burns

      q. Head injury
      r. Smoke inhalation

B. Assessment
1. DYSPNEA, TACHYPNEA, intercostal retractions
2. Cyanosis
3. CRACKLES, RHONCHI
4. Decreased breath sounds
5. Anxiety, restlessness
6. Decreased sensorium

C. Interventions
1. Locate and treat underlying pathology
2. Oxygen therapy: including intubation and mechanical ventilation using positive end-expiratory pressure
3. Monitor vital signs, intake and output, hemodynamic variables, pulse oximetry
4. Bed rest
5. Administer prescribed medications
    a. Antibiotics
    b. Inotropics
    c. Analgesics
    d. Diuretics
    e. Anticoagulants
    f. Steroids
    g. Antianxiety agents
    h. Neuromuscular blocking agents
    i. Surfactant replacement
    j. Antioxidants
    k. Nitric oxide
6. Nutritional support
7. Packed red cell transfusions to maintain hematocrit > 25%

◆ IV. Pulmonary edema

A. Pathophysiology
1. Accumulated fluid in interstitium of lung and alveoli
2. Diminished function of left ventricle causes blood to pool there and in left atrium, with blood eventually backing up into pulmonary veins and capillaries
3. Imbalance of pulmonary capillary hydrostatic pressure, capillary oncotic pressure, capillary permeability, and lymphatic drainage causes fluid infiltration to lungs, impairing gas exchange
4. Chronic or acute
5. May result from a cardiac origin
    a. Atherosclerosis
    b. Myocardial infarction

    c. Myocarditis

    d. Valvular disease

    e. Overload of I.V. fluids

    f. Heart failure

  6. Noncardiac origin

    a. ARDS

    b. Severe neurologic injury

    c. High altitudes

B. Assessment

  1. Dyspnea, tachypnea, ORTHOPNEA; crackles, wheezing, rhonchi

  2. Paroxysmal cough

  3. Blood-tinged, frothy sputum

  4. Agitation, restlessness

  5. Chest pain

  6. Tachycardia

  7. Cold, clammy skin

  8. Diastolic third heart sound gallop

  9. Cyanosis

  10. Decreasing blood pressure

  11. Confusion, stupor

C. Interventions

  1. Administer oxygen as needed, including intubation and mechanical ventilation; continuous positive airway pressure

  2. Bed rest: high Fowler's position, with leg dangling over side of bed

  3. Monitor vital signs, intake and output, hemodynamic variables, laboratory values, ABG levels, pulse oximetry, ECG, pulmonary artery pressures

  4. Diet: Low-sodium, fluid restriction

  5. Administer prescribed medications

    a. Diuretics

    b. Vasodilators

    c. Inotropics

    d. Digitalis glycosides

    e. Nitrates

    f. Analgesics (morphine sulfate)

    g. Antianxiety agents

    h. Bronchodilators

  6. Daily weights

  7. Phlebotomy or plasmapheresis

◆ V. Cor pulmonale

A. Pathophysiology

  1. Hypertrophy and dilation of right ventricle develop secondary to a disease affecting structure or function of the lungs or its vasculature

    2. Hypoxia, constriction of pulmonary blood vessels, and obstruction of pulmonary blood flow lead to increased pulmonary resistance and pulmonary hypertension

    3. Pulmonary hypertension increases the heart's workload; right ventricle hypertrophies to force blood through lungs

    4. Occurs as a result of various chronic disorders of the lungs, pulmonary vasculature, chest wall, and respiratory control center

       a. Chronic obstructive pulmonary disease (COPD)

       b. Bronchial asthma

       c. Vasculitis or connective tissue disease

       d. Pulmonary emboli

       e. Kyphoscoliosis

       f. Muscular dystrophy

       g. Obesity

       h. Pulmonary hypertension

B. Assessment

    1. Early stages

       a. Chronic productive cough

       b. Exertional dyspnea

       c. Wheezing respirations

       d. Fatigue and weakness

    2. Progressive stage

       a. Dyspnea, tachypnea, orthopnea; cyanosis

       b. Dependent edema

       c. Enlarged, tender liver; splenomegaly

       d. Hepatojugular reflux, jugular vein distension

       e. Tachycardia

       f. Decreased CO

C. Interventions

    1. Bed rest

    2. Monitor vital signs, intake and output, hemodynamic variables, ECG

    3. Administer oxygen and medications as prescribed

       a. Digitalis glycosides (if atrial fibrillation present)

       b. Antibiotics

       c. Vasodilators

       d. Anticoagulants

       e. Diuretics

    4. Low-sodium diet with fluid restriction

◆ VI. Atelectasis

A. Pathophysiology

    1. Incomplete expansion of lobules (clusters of alveoli) or lung segments, which may result in partial or complete lung collapse

2. Unoxygenated blood passes through collapsed lung areas unchanged, resulting in hypoxemia
3. Chronic or acute
4. Common causes
   a. Bronchial occlusion by mucus plugs
   b. Occlusion by foreign bodies
   c. Upper abdominal or thoracic surgery
   d. Bronchogenic carcinoma
   e. Inflammatory lung disease
   f. Surfactant disruption

B. Assessment
1. Dyspnea: severe with massive collapse
2. Tachypnea
3. Anxiety
4. Cyanosis
5. Tachycardia
6. Substernal or intercostal retractions
7. Mediastinal shift
8. Elevation of the ipsilateral hemidiaphragm
9. Diminished or bronchial breath sounds

C. Interventions
1. Incentive spirometry
2. Frequent coughing and deep-breathing exercises, ambulation
3. Chest percussion and postural drainage
4. Bronchoscopy
5. Bronchodilators, nebulizers
6. Surgery or radiation therapy (for obstructing neoplasms)
7. Monitor respirations and pulse oximetry

◆ VII. Pneumothorax

A. Pathophysiology
1. Increased tension in the pleural cavity, caused by an increased amount of air between the visceral and parietal pleurae
   a. Causes the lung to progressively collapse
   b. Total lung capacity decreases
   c. V/Q imbalance develops, leading to hypoxemia
2. Open
   a. "Sucking wound"
   b. Atmospheric air (positive pressure) flows directly into pleural cavity (negative pressure)
3. Closed
   a. Blunt trauma
   b. Penetrating: if communication between the atmosphere and pleural space seals itself off

    c. Air enters the pleural space from within the lung, causing increased pleural pressure, preventing lung expansion

4. Hemothorax: accumulation of blood in pleural cavity
5. Spontaneous
    a. Closed
    b. Primary: idiopathic
    c. Secondary: related to a specific disease
    d. Rupture of subpleural bleb at lung surface; causes air leakage into pleural space
5. Tension
    a. Spontaneous or traumatic
    b. Injury permits air to enter but not leave pleural space
    c. Rapid increase in pressure within chest with compression atelectasis of unaffected lung
       (1) Shifts mediastinum to opposite side
       (2) Compression of venae cavae results in decreased venous return and decreased CO
6. Causes
    a. Penetrating injury
    b. Blunt trauma
    c. Insertion of a central line
    d. Barotrauma
    e. Thoracic surgery
    f. Thoracentesis
    g. Pleural or transbronchial biopsy

CLINICAL ALERT

B. Assessment
1. Sudden, sharp, pleuritic pain exacerbated by chest movement, breathing, and coughing
2. Asymmetric chest wall movement
3. Dyspnea, tachypnea; tachycardia, hypotension
4. Cyanosis
5. Respiratory distress
6. Absent or decreased breath sounds on affected side, hyperresonance on affected side, decreased tactile fremitus
7. Chest rigidity
8. Subcutaneous emphysema, neck vein distention
9. Mediastinal shift and tracheal deviation to the opposite side
10. Decreased CO and signs and symptoms of shock

C. Interventions
1. Chest tube insertion
2. Bed rest
3. Monitor vital signs, pulse oximetry, ABG levels
4. Administer oxygen
5. Aspiration of air with large-bore needle attached to a syringe

TEACHING TIPS
Patient with pneumothorax

Be sure to include the following topics in your teaching plan for the patient with pneumothorax:
1. Know signs and symptoms of recurrence and report these immediately to the doctor.
2. Plan activities of daily living to allow adequate rest periods.
3. Obtain immunizations against influenza and pneumococcal pneumonia.
4. Avoid crowds or individuals with colds or other respiratory tract infections.
5. Stop smoking.

6. Thoracoscopy or open thoracotomy
7. Pleurectomy
8. Treatment of underlying pulmonary disease
9. Spontaneous: smoking cessation, avoidance of high altitudes and scuba diving (for additional teaching tips, see *Patient with pneumothorax*)
10. Serial chest X-rays
11. Injection of sclerosing agent into pleural space

◆ VIII. Pneumonia

A. Pathophysiology
1. An acute inflammation of the lung parenchyma and interstitium that often impairs gas exchange
2. Three classifications
   a. Origin: bacterial, viral, fungal, or protozoal (uncommon)
   b. Location
      (1) Bronchopneumonia involves distal airways and alveoli
      (2) Lobular pneumonia, part of a lobe
      (3) Lobar pneumonia, an entire lobe
   c. Type
      (1) Primary: inhalation or aspiration of a pathogen
      (2) Secondary: follows lung damage from a noxious chemical, insult, or hematogenous spread of bacteria
      (3) Aspiration: inhalation of foreign matter
3. Bacterial
   a. Infection triggers alveolar inflammation and edema, producing an area of low ventilation and normal perfusion
   b. Capillaries become more permeable, allowing red blood cells and proteins to leave capillary
   c. Interstitium and alveoli fill with blood and exudate, resulting in atelectasis

4. Viral
   a. Virus first attacks bronchiolar epithelial cells, which causes interstitial inflammation and desquamation
   b. Invades bronchial mucous glands and goblet cells then spreads to the alveoli, which fill with blood and fluid
5. Aspiration
   a. Inhalation of gastric juices or hydrocarbons triggers inflammatory changes and inactivates surfactant over a large area
   b. Decreased surfactant leads to alveolar collapse
   c. Acidic gastric juices may damage airways and alveoli
6. Predisposing factors
   a. Chronic illness and debilitation
   b. Cancer
   c. Abdominal and thoracic surgery
   d. Atelectasis
   e. Colds or other viral respiratory infections
   f. Influenza
   g. Smoking
   h. Malnutrition
   i. Alcoholism
   j. Sickle cell disease
   k. Tracheostomy
   l. Antibiotic therapy
   m. Diabetes mellitus
   n. Chronic bronchitis
      Immunosuppression

B. Assessment and interventions (see *Types of pneumonia,* pages 56 and 57, for specific assessment findings and interventions)

◆ IX. Pulmonary embolism

A. Pathophysiology
   1. Obstruction of pulmonary arterial bed by a dislodged thrombus or foreign substance
   2. Thrombus formation arises from vascular wall damage, venostasis, or hypercoaguability of the blood
   3. Trauma, clot dissolution, sudden muscle spasm, intravascular pressure changes, or a change in peripheral blood flow can cause the thrombus to loosen or fragment and float to the heart's right side and enter the lungs through the pulmonary artery
   4. Occluded pulmonary artery then prevents alveoli from producing enough surfactant to maintain alveolar integrity; alveoli collapse and atelectasis develops
   5. An enlarged embolus may clog most or all pulmonary vessels and cause death

Types of pneumonia

TYPE	SIGNS AND SYMPTOMS	INTERVENTIONS
VIRAL **Influenza** **(prognosis poor** **even with** **treatment; 50%** **mortality)**	• Cough (initially nonproductive; later, purulent sputum), marked cyanosis, dyspnea, high fever, chills, substernal pain and discomfort, moist crackles, frontal headache, myalgia • Death results from cardiopulmonary collapse.	• Supportive: for respiratory failure, endotracheal intubation and ventilator assistance; for fever, hypothermia blanket or antipyretics; for influenza A, amantadine or rimantadine
Adenovirus **(insidious** **onset; generally** **affects young** **adults)**	• Sore throat, fever, cough, chills, malaise, small amounts of mucoid sputum, retrosternal chest pain, anorexia, rhinitis, adenopathy, scattered crackles, and rhonchi	• Treat signs and symptoms only. • Mortality low; usually clears with no residual effects
Respiratory **syncytial virus** **(most prevalent** **in infants and** **children)**	• Listlessness, irritability, tachypnea with retraction of intercostal muscles, slight sputum production, fine moist crackles, fever, severe malaise, and possibly cough or croup	• Supportive: humidified air, oxygen, antimicrobials commonly given until viral etiology confirmed, aerosolized ribavirin • Complete recovery in 1 to 3 weeks
Cytomegalovirus	• Difficult to distinguish from other nonbacterial pneumonias • Fever, cough, shaking chills, dyspnea, cyanosis, weakness, and diffuse crackles • Occurs in neonates as devastating multisystemic infection; in normal adults, resembles mononucleosis; in immunocompromised hosts, varies from clinically inapparent to devastating infection	• Generally, benign and self-limiting in mononucleosis-like form • Supportive: adequate hydration and nutrition, oxygen therapy, bed rest • In immunosuppressed patients, disease is more severe and may be fatal; ganciclovir or foscarnet treatment warranted
BACTERIAL ***Streptococcus*** **(*Streptococcus*** ***pneumoniae*)**	• Sudden onset of a single, shaking chill, and sustained temperature of 102° to 104° F (38.9° to 40° C); commonly preceded by upper respiratory tract infection	• Antimicrobial therapy: penicillin G (or erythromycin, if patient is allergic to penicillin) for 7 to 10 days. Such therapy begins after obtaining culture specimen but without waiting for results. • Pneumococcal vaccination
Klebsiella	• Fever and recurrent chills; cough producing rusty, bloody, viscous sputum (currant jelly); cyanosis of lips and nail beds due to hypoxemia; shallow, grunting respirations • Common in patients with chronic alcoholism, pulmonary disease, or diabetes	• Antimicrobial therapy: an aminoglycoside and a cephalosporin

Types of pneumonia (continued)

TYPE	SIGNS AND SYMPTOMS	INTERVENTIONS
BACTERIAL *Staphylococcus*	• Temperature of 102° to 104° F (38.9° to 40° C), recurrent shaking chills, bloody sputum, dyspnea, tachypnea, and hypoxemia • Should be suspected with viral illness, such as influenza or measles, and in patients with cystic fibrosis	• Antimicrobial therapy: nafcillin or oxacillin for 14 days if staphylococci are penicillinase producing • Supportive: chest tube drainage of empyema
Haemophilus influenzae	• Fever, cough, purulent sputum; usually of several days duration • Prevalent in patients with preexisting lung conditions such as chronic obstructive pulmonary disease (COPD)	• Antimicrobial therapy: erythromycin or tetracycline; clarithromycin or azithromycin if there is an intolerance of erythromycin • Patients with COPD or bronchiectasis or over age 60 should receive a second-generation cephalosporin, trimethoprin-sulfa-methoxazole, or a beta-lactam or beta-lactamase inhibitor with or without a macrolide
PROTOZOAN *Pneumocystis carinii*	• Occurs in immunocompromised persons • Dyspnea and nonproductive cough • Anorexia, weight loss, and fatigue • Low-grade fever	• Antimicrobial therapy: co-trimoxazole or pentamidine by I.V. or inhalation • Supportive: oxygen, improved nutrition, mechanical ventilation
ASPIRATION **Results from vomiting and aspiration of gastric or oropharyngeal contents into trachea and lungs**	• Noncardiogenic pulmonary edema may follow damage to respiratory epithelium from contact with stomach acid. • Crackles, dyspnea, cyanosis, hypotension, and tachycardia • May be subacute pneumonia with cavity formation, or lung abscess may occur if foreign body is present	• Antimicrobial therapy: penicillin G or clindamycin • Supportive: oxygen therapy, suctioning, coughing, deep breathing, adequate hydration

6. Predisposing factors
   a. Long-term immobility
   b. Chronic pulmonary disease
   c. Heart failure or atrial fibrillation
   d. Thrombophlebitis
   e. Autoimmune hemolytic anemia
   f. Recent surgery; childbirth
   g. Lower-extremity fractures or surgery
   h. Vascular injury
   i. Oral contraceptives

    j. Obesity

    k. Advanced age

B. Assessment

  1. Dyspnea, tachypnea

  2. Anginal or pleuritic chest pain

  3. Tachycardia

  4. Productive cough, hemoptysis

  5. Pleural effusion

  6. Pleural friction rub

  7. Restlessness, apprehension

  8. Signs and symptoms of acute right ventricular failure and hypotension

  9. Sudden collapse without signs of shock

C. Interventions

  1. Prevention; attention to those at high risk

  2. Monitor vital signs, respiratory status, ABG levels

  3. Administer oxygen and prescribed medications

    a. Anticoagulants, antiplatelet agents

    b. Fibrinolytics, thrombolytics

    c. Vasopressors

    d. Antibiotics (septic emboli)

    e. Analgesics

  4. Vena caval ligation, plication, clipping; insertion of intraluminal filters in inferior vena cava just below renal veins

  5. Embolectomy

◆ X. Emphysema

A. Pathophysiology

  1. Abnormal, permanent enlargement of the acini accompanied by destruction of the terminal bronchioles and alveolar walls

  2. Caused by recurrent inflammation or absence of enzyme alpha-antitrypsin, or both

  3. Recurrent inflammation is associated with the release of PROTEOLYTIC ENZYMES, such as elastase, which attach structural proteins in walls of terminal bronchioles and alveoli

  4. Irreversible enlargement of the air spaces distal to the terminal bronchioles occurs which destroys the alveolar walls

  5. Elasticity is reduced

    a. Fibrous and muscular tissue loss occurs, making lungs less compliant

    b. Terminal airways and alveoli collapse on expiration, trapping air

  6. Predisposing factors

    a. Smoking

    b. Recurrent respiratory infections

    c. Pollution

B. Assessment
1. Exertional dyspnea; progressive, constant, severe; hyperventilation
2. Barrel-shaped chest from lung overdistention (air trapping); increased anteroposterior (AP) diameter
3. Prolonged expiration
4. Decreased breath sounds, hyperresonance
5. Weight loss; cachexia
6. Hypertrophied accessory respiratory muscles

C. Interventions
1. Monitor vital signs, respiratory status, ABG levels, spirometry
2. Administer prescribed medications
   a. Bronchodilators
   b. Antibiotics
   c. Anticholinergics
   d. Steroids
   e. Antianxiety agents
   f. Corticosteroids
3. Chest physiotherapy
4. Avoidance of smoking and air pollution
5. Pulmonary rehabilitation
6. Oxygen therapy
7. Lung reduction surgery, lung transplantation, bullectomy
8. Nutritional support

◆ XI. Chronic bronchitis

A. Pathophysiology
1. Excessive bronchial mucus production causes chronic or recurrent productive cough that persists for at least 3 months over 2 consecutive years (other disease processes absent)
2. Edema of the bronchial structures occurs and may cause airway obstruction
3. Imbalance between ventilation and perfusion occurs
   a. Hypoxemia and hypercarbia develop
   b. Pulmonary vascular resistance increases
4. Predisposing factors
   a. Smoking
   b. Recurrent respiratory infections
   c. Pollution

B. Assessment
1. Chronic cough: very productive, severe
2. Clubbed fingers
3. Dyspnea: intermittent, mild to moderate
4. Cyanosis
5. Prolonged expiratory phase of respirations

6. Wheezes
7. Crackles, rhonchi
8. Peripheral edema
9. Jugular venous distention
10. Hepatomegaly, splenomegaly

C. Interventions
1. Monitor vital signs and respiratory status, ABGs, spirometry
2. Avoid smoking or areas heavy with cigarette smoke
3. Monitor air pollution levels
4. Administer oxygen as prescribed (at no more than 2 to 3 L/minute), including intubation and ventilation if necessary
5. Administer prescribed medications
   a. Bronchodilators
   b. Corticosteroids
   c. Antibiotics
   d. Antianxiety agents
   e. Anticholinergics
6. Avoid exposure to respiratory tract infections
7. Obtain annual influenza immunization
8. Chest physiotherapy
9. Pulmonary rehabilitation
10. Nutritional support
11. Lung reduction surgery, lung transplantation

◆ XII. Tuberculosis

A. Pathophysiology
1. Infectious disease that primarily affects the lungs but can invade other body systems
2. Results from exposure to *Mycobacterium tuberculosis* and sometimes other strains of *Mycobacterium*
   a. Transmission: infected droplets are inhaled and bacilli are deposited in the lungs
   b. Bacilli are ingested by macrophages and travel to the lymph nodes
   c. Macrophages fuse and form epithelioid cell TUBERCLES
   d. Rupture of tubercles contaminates surrounding tissue and may spread bacteria through blood and lymphatic circulation to distant sites
3. May cause massive pulmonary tissue damage with inflammation and tissue necrosis eventually leading to respiratory failure, bronchopleural fistula, hemorrhage, pleural effusion, and pneumonia

B. Assessment
1. Low-grade fever at night, night sweats
2. Productive cough lasting longer than 3 weeks, hemoptysis

TEACHING TIPS
Patient with tuberculosis

Be sure to include the following topics in your teaching plan for the patient with tuberculosis:
1. Emphasize the need for good handwashing.
2. Cover mouth and nose with double-thickness tissue when coughing or sneezing.
3. Instruct the patient and family on the need to take medications as prescribed; arrange for direct observation therapy (DOT).
4. Avoid crowds or individuals with infections.
5. Stop smoking.
6. Maintain good ventilation in living spaces.

    3. Signs and symptoms of airway obstruction from lymph node involvement
    4. Fatigue
    5. Malaise
    6. Dyspnea, orthopnea
    7. Tachycardia
    8. Weight loss, anorexia

C. Interventions
    1. Monitor vital signs, pulse oximetry, cultures
    2. Administer oxygen and medications as prescribed
      a. Isoniazid
      b. Rifampin
      c. Pyrazinamide
      d. Streptomycin
      e. Ethambutol
    3. Bed rest
    4. Chest physiotherapy, postural drainage, incentive spirometry
    5. Maintain infection-control precautions
    6. Directly observed therapy
    7. Provide information about the American Lung Association (for additional teaching tips, see *Patient with tuberculosis*)
    8. Nutritional support

POINTS TO REMEMBER

◆ The respiratory system performs tissue oxygenation and carbon dioxide removal. It consists of upper airways, lower airways, and lungs.

◆ Assessment findings in respiratory disorders include dyspnea, adventitious sounds, sputum, clubbing of fingers, fremitus, crepitus, and a change in patterns and character of respirations.

◆ The stimulus for breathing in emphysema is low PaO_2.

◆ The patient with ARDS, pneumothorax, or pulmonary embolism should be placed in high Fowler's position (if possible).

◆ Cigarette smoking has a profound effect on the adequate function of lung tissue.

STUDY QUESTIONS

To evaluate your understanding of this chapter, answer the following questions in the space provided; then compare your responses with the correct answers in appendix B, pages 289 and 290.

1. What are the possible causes of pulmonary edema? _____

_____

2. What are the types of pneumothorax? _____

_____

3. What are the assessment findings in a patient with pneumonia? _____

_____

4. What is the cause of chronic bronchitis? _____

_____

CRITICAL THINKING AND APPLICATION EXERCISES

1. Observe a pulmonary resection. Prepare an oral presentation describing the procedure and care of the patient.

2. Interview a patient with emphysema. Evaluate the information for possible risk factors and identify ways to modify them.

3. Develop a chart depicting the different types of pneumothorax and list the treatments of each type.

Hematologic Disorders

CHAPTER OVERVIEW

Blood is one of the body's major fluid tissues. Pumped by the heart, it continuously circulates through the blood vessels, carrying vital elements to every part of the body as well as carrying away waste products. These and other functions make the hematologic system a principle factor in maintenance of homeostasis. Because the condition and relative abundance of blood components can provide clues to many hematologic and other disorders, the health care professional should be familiar with blood composition and normal function.

♦ I. Blood components

    A. Plasma
        1. Carries antibodies and nutrients to tissues
        2. Carries wastes away

     3. Fluid characteristics (dependent on protein content)

       a. Osmotic pressure

       b. Viscosity

       c. Suspension

     4. Regulates acid-base balance and immune responses

     5. Accelerates coagulation

     6. Plasma components

       a. Proteins: globulin, albumin, and fibrinogen

       b. Glucose

       c. Lipids

       d. Amino acids

       e. Electrolytes

       f. Pigments

       g. Hormones

B. Erythrocytes (red blood cells [RBCs])

     1. Carry oxygen to the tissues

     2. Remove carbon dioxide from the tissues

     3. Arise in BONE MARROW; production regulated by tissues' demand for oxygen and blood cells' ability to deliver it

     4. Hypoxia stimulates formation and release of ERYTHROPOIETIN (renal hormone), which stimulates the production of RBCs

C. Leukocytes (white blood cells [WBCs])

     1. Participate in inflammatory and immune responses

     2. GRANULAR

       a. Basophils

         (1) May release heparin and histamine

         (2) May participate in delayed allergic reactions

       b. Neutrophils

         (1) Predominant form

         (2) Surround and digest invading organisms and other foreign matter by PHAGOCYTOSIS

       c. Eosinophils

         (1) Defend against parasites

         (2) Participate in allergic reactions

         (3) Fight lung and skin infections

     3. Nongranular

       a. Lymphocytes

         (1) B-lymphocytes (B cells) produce antibodies

         (2) T-lymphocytes (T cells) regulate cell-mediated immunity

       b. Monocytes

         (1) Devour invading organisms by phagocytosis

         (2) Migrate to tissues and develop into MACROPHAGES (important in immune responses)

    c. Plasma cells
      (1) Develop from B cells in tissues
      (2) Produce, store, and release antibodies

D. Thrombocytes (platelets)
  1. Cytoplasmic cells split from cells in bone marrow
  2. Three vital functions
    a. Shrink damaged blood vessels to minimize blood loss
    b. Form hemostatic plugs in injured blood vessels
    c. Provide materials that accelerate blood coagulation (with plasma), especially factor III
  3. When the clot is no longer needed, the fibrin is dissolved or lysed (fibrinolysis)

◆ II. Dyscrasias

A. Types
  1. Qualitative: stem from intrinsic cell abnormalities or plasma component dysfunction
  2. Quantitative: result from increased or decreased cell production or cell destruction

B. Causes
  1. Trauma
  2. Chronic disease
  3. Surgery
  4. Malnutrition
  5. Drugs
  6. Toxins
  7. Radiation
  8. Genetic and congenital defects
  9. Sepsis
  10. Viruses

◆ III. Iron deficiency anemia

A. Pathophysiology
  1. The most common form of anemia
  2. It is caused by an inadequate supply of iron for optimal formation of RBCs, resulting in microcytic cells
  3. Body stores of iron decrease, as do levels of transferrin, which binds with and transports iron
  4. Insufficient body stores of iron lead to a depleted RBC mass
    a. Decreased hemoglobin concentration (hypochromia)
    b. Decreased oxygen-carrying capacity of the blood
  5. May result from
    a. Inadequate dietary intake of iron
    b. Iron malabsorption

    c. Blood loss

    d. Pregnancy

    e. Intravascular HEMOLYSIS-induced hemoglobinuria or paroxysmal nocturnal hemoglobinuria

    f. Mechanical erythrocyte trauma caused by a prosthetic heart valve or umbrella filters (vena caval filters)

B. Assessment

    1. Exertional dyspnea

    2. Fatigue, listlessness

    3. Pallor

    4. Irritability or inability to concentrate

    5. Headache

    6. Susceptibility to infection

    7. Tachycardia

    8. In chronic iron deficiency anemia, signs and symptoms also include

        a. Spoon-shaped, brittle nails

        b. Smooth tongue

        c. Dysphagia

        d. Pica

        e. Vasomotor disturbances

        f. Numbness and tingling of the extremities

        g. Neuralgic pain

C. Interventions

    1. Determine the underlying cause of anemia and treat accordingly

    2. Treatment of choice is an oral preparation of iron or a combination of iron and ascorbic acid (to enhance iron absorption)

    3. Administer parenteral iron

        a. If patient is noncompliant with oral preparation

        b. If there is a need for a higher dose than can be taken orally

        c. If malabsorption prevents adequate iron absorption

        d. If a maximum rate of hemoglobin regeneration is desired

    4. Teach the basics of a nutritionally balanced diet

        a. Red meats, fish, or poultry

        b. Green vegetables

        c. Eggs

        d. Whole wheat products

        e. Iron-fortified bread

        f. Foods high in ascorbic acid

    5. Emphasize the need for prophylactic oral iron to high-risk individuals

        a. Premature or low-birth-weight infants

        b. Children under age 2

        c. Pregnant women

        d. Adolescent girls (for additional teaching tips, see *Patient with iron deficiency anemia*)

TEACHING TIPS
Patient with iron deficiency anemia

Be sure to include the following topics in your teaching plan for the patient with iron deficiency anemia:
1. Increase dietary grains, vegetables, legumes, and nuts.
2. Increase vitamin C intake to enhance iron absorption.
3. Limit intake of tea and coffee, which inhibit iron absorption.
4. Limit use of antacids.
5. If taking a commercial supplement, be aware that they may cause darkening of stools, as well as gastrointestinal discomfort (nausea, diarrhea, heartburn).

♦ IV. Pernicious anemia

A. Pathophysiology
1. Megablastic anemia characterized by decreased gastric production of hydrochloric acid and deficiency of intrinsic factor (essential for vitamin B_{12} absorption)
2. Vitamin B_{12} deficiency inhibits cell growth, particularly RBCs, leading to insufficient and deformed RBCs with poor oxygen-carrying capacity; impairs myelin formation
3. Possible causes
   a. Genetic predisposition suggested due to familial incidence
   b. Immunologically related diseases

B. Assessment
1. Weakness, fatigue
2. Numbness and tingling in the extremities
3. Nausea and vomiting, diarrhea, abdominal pain
4. Neuritis
5. Lack of coordination
6. Irritability
7. Poor memory
8. Shortness of breath, palpitations, chest pain

C. Interventions
1. Parenteral vitamin B_{12} replacement
2. Bed rest until hemoglobin level increases
3. Blood transfusion

♦ V. Polycythemia vera (primary polycythemia)

A. Pathophysiology
1. Chronic, myeloproliferative disorder
2. Characterized by increased RBC mass, leukocytosis, thrombocytosis, and increased hemoglobin concentration, with normal or increased plasma volume

3. Uncontrolled and rapid cellular reproduction and maturation cause proliferation or hyperplasia of all bone marrow cells (panmyelosis)
4. Cause is unknown; probably due to a multipotential stem cell defect

B. Assessment
1. Hypervolemia, hyperviscosity
2. Feeling of fullness in the head, headache, dizziness; inability to concentrate
3. Thrombosis of smaller vessels
4. Ruddy cyanosis
5. Clubbing of digits
6. Hemorrhage
7. Hypertension
8. Night sweats
9. Weight loss
10. Palpable spleen

C. Interventions
1. Phlebotomy
2. Apheresis
3. Myelosuppressive therapy: radioactive phosphorus or chemotherapeutic agents
4. Monitor vital signs, laboratory values
5. Observe for signs and symptoms of abnormal bleeding or clotting or both

♦ VI. Thrombocytopenia

A. Pathophysiology
1. Deficiency of circulating platelets
   a. Decreased or defective production of platelets in the marrow (leukemia, aplastic anemia)
   b. Increased destruction outside the marrow caused by an underlying disorder (liver cirrhosis, disseminated intravascular coagulation [DIC], idiopathic thrombocytopenic purpura [ITP])
   c. Sequestration (hypersplenism, hypothermia)
   d. Platelet loss (hemorrhage)
2. Causes
   a. Congenital
   b. Acquired: drugs, radiation
   c. Idiopathic: occurs in children (unknown pathology)

B. Assessment
1. Sudden onset of petechiae or ecchymoses in the skin
2. Bleeding from any mucous membrane or into any organ or potential space
3. Malaise
4. Fatigue

5. Large blood-filled bullae in the mouth

C. Interventions
1. Monitor vital signs and laboratory tests
2. Administer prescribed medications
   a. Corticosteroids
   b. Immune globulin
3. Treat underlying cause
4. Avoid I.M. injections, enemas, and rectal temperatures
5. Monitor for signs of bleeding: petechiae, ecchymoses, surgical or GI bleeding, menorrhagia, cerebral hemorrhage
6. Platelet transfusion
7. Splenectomy

◆ VII. Disseminated intravascular coagulation

A. Pathophysiology
1. Clotting and hemorrhage occur in the vascular system at the same time
2. Also called consumption coagulopathy or defibrination syndrome
3. Excess fibrin is formed and becomes trapped in the microvasculature along with platelets, causing clots
4. Blood flow to tissues decreases, causing acidemia, blood stasis, and tissue hypoxia; organ failure may result
5. Both fibrinolysis and antithrombotic mechanisms lead to anticoagulation
6. Platelets and coagulation factors are consumed and massive hemorrhage may ensue
7. Usually develops in association with three pathologic processes
   a. Damage to endothelium
   b. Release of tissue thromboplastin
   c. Activation of factor X (see *Three mechanisms of DIC,* page 70)
8. Possible causes
   a. Infection
   b. Obstetric complications
   c. Neoplastic disease
   d. Disorders that produce necrosis
   e. Other conditions: shock, drug reactions, cardiac arrest, surgery necessitating cardiopulmonary bypass, adult respiratory distress syndrome (ARDS), pulmonary embolism, massive trauma

B. Assessment
1. Abnormal bleeding without history of serious hemorrhagic disorder
2. Cutaneous oozing
3. Petechiae or blood blisters
4. Bleeding from surgical or I.V. sites
5. Bleeding from GI tract

Three mechanisms of DIC

However disseminated intravascular coagulation (DIC) begins, accelerated clotting (characteristic of DIC) usually results in excess thrombin, which in turn causes fibrinolysis with excess fibrin formation and fibrin degradation products (FDP), activation of fibrin-stabilizing factor (factor XIII), consumption of platelet and clotting factors and, eventually, hemorrhage.

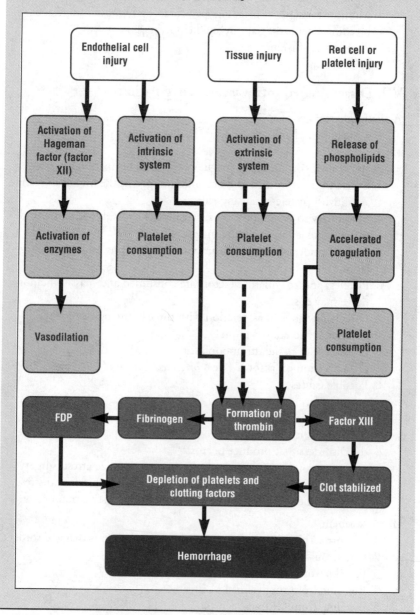

      6. Cyanosis of extremities

      7. Severe muscle, back, abdominal, and chest pain

      8. Nausea and vomiting

      9. Seizures, coma

    10. Oliguria

    11. Shock

    12. ARDS

C. Interventions

    1. Monitor vital signs, laboratory values

    2. Administer fresh frozen plasma, platelets, packed RBCs, or cryoprecipitate as prescribed

    3. Treat underlying disorder

    4. Administer heparin in early stages and as last resort in hemorrhage (controversial)

    5. Bleeding precautions

◆ VIII. Idiopathic thrombocytopenic purpura

A. Pathophysiology

    1. ITP results from immunologic platelet destruction secondary to formation of platelet antibodies

    2. Circulating immunoglobulin G molecules react with host platelets, which are destroyed by phagocytosis in the spleen or liver

    3. Acute ITP

      a. Usually affects children ages 2 to 6

      b. Commonly follows viral infection or immunization with a live vaccine

      c. Bleeding is sudden

    4. Chronic ITP

      a. Linked with immunologic disorders

      b. Bleeding is insidious (usual adult presentation)

B. Assessment

    1. Nosebleed

    2. Oral bleeding

    3. Purpura

    4. Petechiae

    5. Excessive menstruation

    6. Splenomegaly

C. Interventions

    1. Monitor vital signs, laboratory values

    2. Administer prescribed medications

      a. Corticosteroids

      b. Immune globulin

      c. Immunosuppressants

    3. Plasmapheresis or platelet APHERESIS with transfusion

    4. Splenectomy

POINTS TO REMEMBER

♦ Blood performs vital transportation, regulation, and protection functions.

♦ I.M. injections, enemas, and rectal temperatures should be avoided in patients with bleeding tendencies.

♦ Blood vessels, platelets, and coagulation factors help blood to clot. When the clot is no longer needed, it must be lysed, which is done by fibrinolysis.

STUDY QUESTIONS

To evaluate your understanding of this chapter, answer the following questions in the space provided; then compare your responses with the correct answers in appendix B, page 290.

1. What is a vital function of platelets? _____

_____

2. What are three possible treatments for thrombocytopenia? _____

_____

3. What is the pathophysiology of DIC? _____

_____

4. What is the pathophysiology of ITP?_____

_____

CRITICAL THINKING AND APPLICATION EXERCISES

1. Follow a patient with a hematologic disorder from admission through discharge. Develop a patient-specific plan of care, including any needs for follow-up and home care.

2. Develop a chart comparing the major drug classes used for treating bleeding disorders.

3. Identify the arguments for and against using heparin in the treatment of DIC.

4. Develop a teaching plan for adolescent girls for preventing or improving iron deficiency anemia.

5. Develop a nutritional teaching plan for vegetarian patients.

Neurologic Disorders

LEARNING OBJECTIVES

After studying this chapter, you should be able to:

♦ Identify the structures of the neurologic system.

♦ Describe how the neurologic system works.

♦ Describe the psychosocial impact of nervous system disorders.

♦ Differentiate between modifiable and nonmodifiable risk factors in the development of a nervous system disorder.

♦ List three interventions for a patient with a nervous system disorder.

CHAPTER OVERVIEW

By serving as the body's control and communication center, the nervous system directs every body system and governs all movement, sensation, thought, and emotion. It senses internal and external changes, analyzes and stores this sensory information, makes decisions about it and responds to it: all within a brief time. A thorough assessment is essential to planning and implementing appropriate patient care. Nursing diagnoses focus primarily on self-care deficits, altered cerebral tissue perfusion, and decreased adaptive intracranial capacity.

♦ I. Central nervous system (CNS)

A. Brain: major components
   1. CEREBRUM
      a. Right and left hemispheres; frontal, parietal, temporal, occipital, and limbic lobes
         (1) Controls sensory, motor, auditory, and visual functions
         (2) Location of intellectual, cognitive, judgement, and emotional functions
      b. Basal ganglia
         (1) Controls involuntary motor movements
         (2) Contributes to imitation, modulation, and completion of voluntary movement
      c. Diencephalon
         (1) Relay center for sensory data to and from cerebral cortex in cerebrum
         (2) Responsible for primitive emotional responses
         (3) Distinguishes pleasant stimuli from unpleasant ones
   2. Hypothalamus
      a. Located beneath the thalamus
      b. Autonomic center with connections to the brain, spinal cord, autonomic nervous system, and pituitary gland
      c. Control center for homeostasis; regulates temperature, appetite, blood pressure, breathing, sleep patterns, and peripheral discharges that occur with behavioral and emotional expression
   3. Cerebellum
      a. Beneath the occipital lobe on the dorsal surface of brain stem
      b. Coordinates muscle movements, posture
      c. Maintains equilibrium
   4. Brain stem: three divisions
      a. Midbrain
         (1) Reflex center for cranial nerves III and IV
         (2) Mediates pupillary reflexes, eye movement, and lid elevation
      b. Pons
         (1) Helps regulate respirations
         (2) Reflex center for cranial nerves V through VIII
         (3) Mediates chewing, taste, saliva secretion, hearing, and equilibrium
         (4) Area for large number of nerve fibers to and from cerebellum
      c. Medulla oblongata
         (1) Influences cardiac, respiratory, and vasomotor functions
         (2) Center for vomiting, coughing and hiccuping reflexes
   5. Upper motor neurons
      a. Conduct motor impulses from brain to spinal cord
      b. Form two systems

(1) Pyramidal system (corticospinal tract): responsible for fine, skilled movements of skeletal muscles

(2) Extrapyramidal system (extracorticospinal tract): controls gross motor movements

6. Lower motor neurons (spinal motor neurons): conduct impulses that originate in upper motor neurons to the muscles

B. Spinal cord

1. Functions as a two-way conducting pathway between the cerebrum, cerebellum, and brain stem and the peripheral nervous system

2. Gray matter consists mostly of neuron cell bodies

3. White matter consists of myelinated nerve fibers grouped into tracts

   a. Sensory (ascending) tracts: carry impulses up the spinal cord to the brain

   b. Motor (descending) tracts: carry impulses down the spinal cord and continue to peripheral nervous system

4. White and gray matter contain numerous reflex centers

C. Protection

1. Brain, brain stem, and cerebellum protected by bony skull and cervical vertebrae

2. Spinal cord protected by vertebral column

3. Both brain and spinal cord also protected by three membranes

   a. Dura mater

   (1) Outermost covering

   (2) Provides support and protection

   (3) Adheres to skull and vertebral column

   (4) Subdural space is a potential space

   b. Arachnoid membrane

   (1) Hugs the brain and spinal cord

   (2) Lies under the dura mater

   (3) Subarachnoid space is filled with cerebrospinal fluid (CSF) and serves as a pathway to large arteries

   c. Pia mater: adheres to every contour of brain and spinal cord

D. Blood supply

1. Brain and spinal cord supplied by two major arterial systems and their branches

   a. Internal carotid

   b. Vertebral basilar

   c. These two systems connect at the base of the brain in the circle of Willis

2. Venous drainage for brain provided by internal jugular vein

◆ II. Peripheral nervous system

A. Autonomic nervous system
1. Helps regulate the body's internal environment through involuntary control of organ systems
2. Divided into two antagonistic systems that balance each other to support homeostasis
   a. Sympathetic nervous system
      (1) Active in fight-or-flight situations (stress)
      (2) Catabolic in nature
      (3) Primary neurotransmitter is norepinephrine
   b. Parasympathetic nervous system
      (1) Controls "maintenance and housekeeping" functions in non-stress situations
      (2) Anabolic in nature
      (3) Primary neurotransmitter is acetylcholine

B. Spinal nerves (32 or more pairs) attached to the spinal cord by two roots
1. Anterior or ventral root
   a. Consists of motor fibers
   b. Relays impulses from the spinal cord to the glands and muscles
2. Posterior or dorsal root
   a. Consists of sensory fibers
   b. Relays information from receptors to the spinal cord

C. Cranial nerves (12 pairs, usually designated by Roman numerals)
1. Olfactory (I)
2. Optic (II)
3. Oculomotor (III)
4. Trochlear (IV)
5. Trigeminal (V)
6. Abducens (VI)
7. Facial (VII)
8. Vestibulocochlear (VIII)
9. Glossopharyngeal (IX)
10. Vagus (X)
11. Spinal accessory (XI)
12. Hypoglossal (XII)

◆ III. Headache

A. Pathophysiology
1. Vascular or muscle contraction, or a combination (migraine headaches are vascular)
2. Most common patient complaint

3. Possible causes
   a. Tension from emotional stress, fatigue, menstruation, environmental stimuli
   b. Glaucoma
   c. Inflammation of eyes or mucosa of the nasal or paranasal sinuses
   d. Diseases of the scalp, teeth, extracranial arteries
   e. Muscle spasms of the face, neck or shoulders
   f. Cervical arthritis
   g. Vasodilators
   h. Systemic disease
   i. Hypoxia
   j. Hypertension
   k. Head trauma and tumor
   l. Intracranial bleeding, abscess aneurysm, arteriovenous malformation (AVM)
   m. Increased intracranial pressure

B. Assessment
   1. Dull, persistent ache
   2. Tender spots on the head and neck
   3. Tightness around the head ("hatband" distribution) with muscle contraction; unilateral throbbing in migraine accompanied by nausea and photophobia
   4. Pain may be severe and unrelenting; if caused by intracranial bleeding, narcotics will be ineffective
   5. Nausea and vomiting

C. Interventions
   1. Identify triggers and remove or avoid if possible
   2. Administer prescribed medications
      a. Analgesics, nonsteroidal anti-inflammatory drugs
      b. Tranquilizers, antidepressants
      c. Muscle relaxants
      d. Ergotamine preparations
      e. Sumatriptan
      f. Prophylaxis for migraine with beta blockers or calcium channel blockers
   3. Treatment of causative factors
   4. Psychotherapy, biofeedback, relaxation therapies

◆ IV. Epilepsy

A. Pathophysiology
   1. Chronic brain disorder characterized by recurrent seizures; also known as "seizure disorder"
   2. Paroxysmal event associated with abnormal electrical discharges of neurons in the brain that may trigger a convulsive movement, an in-

terruption of sensation, an alteration in level of consciousness (LOC), or a combination of these signs and symptoms

3. A group of neurons may lose afferent stimulation and function as an epileptogenic focus; are hypersensitive, are easily activated, and fire abnormally

   a. The electronic balance at the neuronal level is altered, causing neuronal membranes to become susceptible to activation

   b. Increased permeability of the cytoplasmic membranes allows hypersensitive neurons to fire abnormally; activated by hyperthermia, hypoglycemia, hyponatremia, hypoxia, or repeated sensory stimulation

   c. Once the intensity of a seizure discharge has progressed sufficiently, it spreads to adjacent brain areas; excitement feeds back from the primary focus and to other parts of the brain

   d. Discharges become less frequent until they stop

4. Possible causes

   a. Idiopathic (approximately 50% of patients)

   b. Genetic abnormalities

   c. Perinatal abnormalities

   d. Brain tumors

   e. Infection

   f. Traumatic injury

   g. Cerebrovascular accident (CVA)

   h. Ingestion of toxins

   i. Fever

B. Assessment

1. Recurring partial seizures

   a. Simple partial motor type: stiffening or jerking in one extremity, accompanied by a tingling sensation in the same area

   b. Simple partial sensory type: perceptual distortion

   c. Complex partial: signs and symptoms vary; includes purposeless behavior (automatisms); often referred to as "psychomotor" or "temporal lobe" seizures

2. Recurring generalized seizures

   a. Absence (petit mal): generalized; brief change in LOC; may progress to tonic-clonic

   b. Myoclonic (bilateral massive epileptic myoclonus): generalized; brief, involuntary muscular jerks of the body or extremities

   c. Generalized tonic-clonic (grand mal): loud cry followed by loss of consciousness; body stiffens (tonic phase) then alternates between episodes of muscular spasm and relaxation (clonic phase)

   d. Akinetic or atonic: general loss of postural tone and temporary loss of consciousness

   e. Status epilepticus: continuous seizure state; respiratory distress may occur

C. Interventions
  1. Document seizure characteristics and frequency
  2. Monitor vital signs and neurologic status
  3. Maintain safety of patient's environment
  4. Administer anticonvulsant medications as ordered
  5. Surgical removal of a demonstrated focal lesion or underlying problem; hemispherectomy

◆ **V. Cerebrovascular accident (brain attack)**

A. Pathophysiology
  1. Sudden impairment of cerebral circulation in one or more of the blood vessels supplying the brain; interrupts or diminishes oxygen supply, causing serious damage or necrosis in brain
  2. Classifications
    a. Transient ischemic attack
      (1) Least severe
      (2) Temporary interruption in blood flow, lasting less than 24 hours
      (3) Usually in carotid and vertebrobasilar arteries (see *Transient ischemic attack,* page 80)
    b. Progressive stroke or "stroke-in-evolution"
      (1) Slight neurologic deficit
      (2) Worsens in 1 to 2 days
    c. Completed stroke: most severe; causes maximum neurologic deficits at onset
  3. Major causes
    a. Thrombosis
      (1) Most common
      (2) Obstruction in extracerebral or intracerebral vessels
      (3) Causes congestion and edema in the affected vessel as well as ischemia in the brain tissue supplied by the vessel
    b. Embolism
      (1) Occlusion caused by a fragmented clot, tumor, fat, bacteria, or air
      (2) Cuts off circulation causing necrosis and edema
    c. Hemorrhage
      (1) Sudden rupture of a cerebral artery, aneurysm, or AVM
      (2) Blood supply diminished to the area served by the artery
      (3) Blood also accumulates deep within the brain, compromising neural tissue
  4. Risk factors for CVA
    a. Age
    b. Race: black men at higher risk than other populations
    c. Hypertension

Transient ischemic attack

A transient ischemic attack (TIA) is a recurrent episode of neurologic deficit, lasting from seconds to hours, that clears within 12 to 24 hours. It's usually considered a warning sign of an impending thrombotic cerebrovascular accident (CVA). In fact, TIAs have been reported in 50% to 80% of patients who have had a cerebral infarction from such thrombosis. The age of onset varies. Incidence rises dramatically after age 50 and is highest among blacks and men.

Causes
In TIA, microemboli released from a thrombus probably temporarily interrupt blood flow, especially in the small distal branches of the arterial tree in the brain. Small spasms in those arterioles may impair blood flow and also precede TIA. Predisposing factors are the same as for thrombotic CVAs. The most distinctive characteristics of TIAs are the transient duration of neurologic deficits and complete return of normal function. The signs and symptoms of TIA easily correlate with the location of the affected artery. These signs and symptoms include double vision, speech deficits (slurring or thickness), unilateral blindness, staggering or uncoordinated gait, unilateral weakness or numbness, falling because of weakness in the legs, and dizziness.

Treatment
During an active TIA, treatment aims to prevent a completed stroke and consists of aspirin or anticoagulants to minimize the risk of thrombosis. After or between attacks, preventive treatment includes carotid endarterectomy or cerebral microvascular bypass.

      d. Atherosclerosis
      e. Arrhythmias
      f. Obesity
      g. Smoking
      h. Oral contraceptive use
      i. Surgery

B. Assessment
  1. Signs and symptoms dependent on brain area that is affected
    a. CVA in the left hemisphere produces signs and symptoms on the right side of the body; usually results in some dysphasia; depression
    b. CVA in the right hemisphere produces signs and symptoms on the left side of the body; usually results in spatial problems, orientation problems, and problems with body boundaries ("neglect" syndrome, impetuousness, unawareness of limitations)
    c. CVA that damages cranial nerves produces signs and symptoms on the same side as the hemorrhage

    2. Altered LOC

    3. Change in motor function and muscle strength

    4. Visual field loss or disturbances

    5. Dysphasia or dysphagia

    6. Personality changes; confusion, depression

    7. Neglect syndrome

    8. Spatial disorientation

C. Interventions

    1. Monitor vital signs, neurologic status

    2. Administer prescribed medications

      a. Anticonvulsants

      b. Stool softeners

      c. Corticosteroids

      d. Anticoagulants

      e. Analgesics

      f. Thrombolytic agents

      g. Antiarrhythmics

    3. Physical therapy, speech therapy, occupational therapy

    4. Craniotomy

    5. Endarterectomy

    6. Extracranial to intracranial bypass

    7. Ventricular shunt

♦ VI. Meningitis

A. Pathophysiology

    1. Inflammation of brain and spinal cord MENINGES; usually the arachnoid membrane and the pia mater

    2. Possible causes

      a. Bacterial: bacteria enter the subarachnoid space, usually after invading and infecting another region of the body

      b. Viral (enteroviruses, arbovirus)

        (1) Called aseptic viral meningitis

        (2) A benign syndrome with mild signs and symptoms

        (3) Self-limiting

      c. Protozoal infection

      d. Fungal infection

      e. Penetrating or non penetrating skull fracture

      f. Lumbar puncture

      g. Ventricular shunting procedures

      h. Herpes simplex, mumps, leukemia

      i. Cranial surgery

B. Assessment

    1. Nuchal rigidity

    2. Exaggerated and symmetrical deep tendon reflexes

3. Opisthotonos (spasm in which the back and extremities arch back-ward so that the body rests on the head and heels)
4. Positive BRUDZINSKI'S SIGN
5. Positive KERNIG'S SIGN
6. Fever, chills
7. Headache
8. Vomiting
9. Photophobia
10. Seizures
11. Focal neurologic deficits

C. Interventions
1. Monitor vital signs
2. Administer prescribed medications
   a. I.V. antibiotics
   b. Mannitol
   c. I.V. anticonvulsants
   d. Acetaminophen
   e. Corticosteroids
3. Bed rest
4. Hypothermia
5. Fluid therapy
6. Treatment of coexisting condition
7. Management of increased intracranial pressure

♦ VII. Encephalitis

A. Pathophysiology
1. Severe inflammation of the brain parenchyma; usually viral, but also due to bacteria, fungi, and other organisms
2. Intense lymphocytic infiltration of the brain tissues and lep-tomeninges causes hemorrhage and cerebral edema, degeneration of nerve cells
3. Possible causes
   a. Arbovirus specific to rural areas; enterovirus in urban areas
   b. Herpes simplex virus
   c. Mumps virus
   d. Human immunodeficiency virus (HIV)
   e. Adenoviruses
   f. Rabies virus
   g. Cytomegalovirus
   h. Demyelinating diseases secondary to measles, varicella, rubella, or vaccination

B. Assessment
1. Sudden onset of fever, headache, and vomiting
2. Stiff neck and back

3. Drowsiness; coma (may persist for days or weeks)
4. Facial paralysis, seizures, ataxia
5. Nausea, vomiting
6. Wide variety of neurologic disturbances

C. Interventions
1. Supportive treatment
2. Administer prescribed medications
    a. Anticonvulsants
    b. Glucosteroids
    c. Mannitol
    d. Sedatives
    e. Acetaminophen
    f. Antibiotics (if appropriate)
3. Fluid therapy
4. Management of increased intracranial pressure

♦ VIII. Parkinson's disease

A. Pathophysiology
1. Chronic progressive disease of the basal ganglia (extrapyramidal system) that influences the initiation, modulation, and completion of motor movements
    a. Results in muscle rigidity and involuntary (resting) tremors
    b. One of the most crippling diseases in the United States
2. Reduction of dopamine in the corpus striatum of the basal ganglia upsets the normal balance between the inhibitory dopamine and excitatory acetylcholine neurotransmitters
3. Cells in corpus stratum are inhibited from performing their normal inhibitory function within the CNS
4. Cause usually unknown; some cases result from exposure to toxins

B. Assessment
1. Muscle rigidity: uniform ("lead pipe") or jerky ("cogwheel")
2. Akinesia
    a. Bradykinesia
        (1) Initiating and performing slow motor movements
        (2) Freezing in place
        (3) Difficulty in changing direction or turning
        (4) Small, shuffling steps
    b. Hypokinesia
        (1) Loss of involuntary motor movements (blinking, swinging arms when walking, spontaneous facial expressions)
        (2) Masklike facial expression
    c. Low postural or righting reflexes
3. Resting pill-rolling tremor
4. High-pitched monotone voice

5. Drooling
6. Dysarthria
7. Fatigue
8. Muscle cramps in the legs, neck, and trunk
9. Mood changes
10. MICROGRAPHIA (a sign of Parkinson's disease)
11. Dementia
12. Autonomic system disturbances (such as increased sweating, impotence, urinary incontinence, constipation, orthostatic hypotension)

C. Interventions
1. Administer prescribed medications
    a. Drugs that increase dopamine levels (levodopa, carbidopa, symmetrol, bromocriptine, selegiline)
    b. Anticholinergics
    c. Antihistamines
    d. Tricyclic antidepressants
2. Stereotactic neurosurgery: subthalamotomy, pallidotomy, transplantation of fetal dopaminergic tissue
3. Physical therapy; nutritional support
4. Maintain patient safety: environmental assessment

♦ **IX. Alzheimer's disease**

A. Pathophysiology
1. Chronic progressive degenerative disorder of the cerebral cortex, resulting in progressive decline in memory, judgement, intellectual function, and adaptive ability
2. Affected brain tissue has three distinguishing features
    a. Neurofibrillary tangles formed out of proteins in the neurons
    b. Neuritic plaques
    c. Granulovascular degeneration of neurons
3. Degeneration of neurons, especially in the frontal, parietal, and occipital lobes; causes enlargement of the ventricles
4. Formation of microscopic plaques containing amyloid (exerts neurotoxic effects); later, atrophy of cerebral cortex becomes evident
5. Possible causes
    a. Neurochemical factors: deficiencies in the neurotransmitter acetylcholine, somatostatin, substance P, and norepinephrine
    b. Environmental factors: repeated exposure to aluminum, manganese, silicon, iron
    c. Viral factors: slow-growing CNS viruses
    d. Repeated head trauma
    e. Genetic factors: familial tendencies

TEACHING TIPS
Patient with Alzheimer's disease

Be sure to include the following topics in your teaching plan for the patient with Alzheimer's disease:
1. Perform an environmental assessment of the home to avoid or minimize the risk of injury and wandering.
2. Keep the environment simple and uncluttered; maintain a daily routine.
3. Wear some form of identificaion at all times.
4. Continue participating in social activities in and out of the home as long as possible.
5. Plan activities of daily living to maximize independence.
6. Join a support group.

B. Assessment
   1. Insidious onset
   2. Forgetfulness
   3. Subtle memory loss without loss of social skills or behavior patterns
   4. Difficulty learning and retaining new information
   5. Inability to concentrate
   6. Deterioration in personal hygiene and appearance
   7. Progressive signs and symptoms
      a. Flattened affect
      b. Difficulty with abstract thinking
      c. Progressive difficulty communicating
      d. Repetitive actions
      e. Mood swings, irritability
      f. Nocturnal awakenings
      g. Incontinence
      h. Seizures

C. Interventions
   1. Administer prescribed medications
      a. Cerebral vasodilators
      b. Hyperbaric oxygen
      c. Psychostimulators
      d. Antidepressants
      e. Experimental drugs (such as antioxidants)
      f. Tacrine, donepezil
   2. Offer emotional support to patient and family
   3. Maintain safety of patient
   4. Regular exercise; good nutrition (for additional teaching tips, see *Patient with Alzheimer's disease*)

◆ X. Guillain-Barré syndrome

A. Pathophysiology

1. Acute, rapidly progressive polyneuropathy; potentially fatal
2. Immunologic reaction causes segmental demyelination of the peripheral nerves, preventing normal transmission of electrical impulses along the sensorimotor nerve roots
3. Myelin sheath degenerates for unknown reasons
   a. Inflammation, swelling, and patchy demyelination occurs
   b. Nodes of Ranvier widen
   c. Impulse transmission along the dorsal and ventral nerve roots are impaired
4. Syndrome has three phases
   a. Acute phase: begins when the first definitive sign or symptom develops and ends 1 to 3 weeks later, when no further deterioration is noted
   b. Plateau phase: lasts for several days to 2 weeks
   c. Recovery phase: believed to coincide with remyelination and axonal process regrowth; can last 4 months to 3 years
5. Precise cause unknown; possibly caused by cell-mediated immunologic attack on peripheral nerves following viral infection

B. Assessment

1. Minor febrile illness 10 to 14 days before onset
2. Symmetrical ascending muscle weakness and paralysis: usually in the legs first then in the arms
3. Tingling and numbness
4. Muscle stiffness and pain
5. Sensory loss; loss of position sense; diminished or absent deep tendon reflexes
6. Reduction or loss of functional breathing
7. Autonomic dysfunction (for example, postural hypotension, arrhythmias, facial flushing, urine retention)

C. Interventions

1. Monitor vital signs, neurological status, and respiratory status
2. Administer oxygen as needed, including endotracheal intubation and mechanical ventilation
3. High-dose I.V. immune globulin
4. Plasmapheresis
5. Physical therapy
6. Corticosteroids

◆ XI. Myasthenia gravis

A. Pathophysiology

1. Sporadic, progressive weakness and abnormal fatigue of voluntary skeletal muscles
2. Blood cells and thymus gland produce antibodies that block, destroy, or weaken the acetylcholine receptors that transmit nerve impulses, causing a failure in transmission of nerve impulses at the neuromuscular junction
3. Usually affects muscles in the face, lips, tongue, neck, and throat, but it can affect any muscle group
4. Myasthenic crisis: acute exacerbation that causes severe respiratory distress
5. Cause is unknown; commonly accompanies autoimmune and thyroid disorders

B. Assessment

1. Extreme muscle weakness
2. Fatigue
3. Ptosis
4. Diplopia
5. Difficulty chewing and swallowing
6. Drooping jaw
7. Bobbing head
8. Arm or hand muscle weakness
9. Weakness of respiratory muscles

C. Interventions

1. Monitor vital signs, neurologic status
2. Administer prescribed medications
   a. I.V. immunoglobulin
   b. Anticholinesterases
   c. Corticosteroids and other immunosuppressants
   d. Antineoplastic agents
3. Assess swallow and gag reflexes
4. Provide rest periods; monitor activity tolerance
5. Provide information about the Myasthenia Gravis Foundation
6. Plasmapheresis
7. Thymectomy
8. Provide respiratory support in crisis

◆ XII. Amyotrophic lateral sclerosis

A. Pathophysiology

1. Chronic, progressive motor neuron disease that causes degeneration of anterior horn cells and corticospinal tracts, resulting in muscle atrophy; also called Lou Gehrig's disease

CLINICAL ALERT

2. Possible causes
   a. Slow-acting virus
   b. Nutritional deficiency related to a disturbance in enzyme metabolism
   c. Metabolic interference in nucleic acid production by the nerve fibers
   d. Autoimmune disorders that affect immune complexes in the renal glomerulus and basement membrane
   e. Genetic, familial
3. Precipitating factors include severe stress, trauma, viral infection, and physical exhaustion

B. Assessment
   1. Muscle weakness, spasticity, stiffness, atrophy, fasciculations
   2. Impaired speech
   3. Difficulty chewing and swallowing
   4. Difficulty breathing
   5. Depression; crying spells or inappropriate laughter
   6. Aspiration

C. Interventions
   1. No effective treatment; symptomatic treatment
   2. Implement a rehabilitation program designed to maintain independence as long as possible
   3. Maintain safety of patient; environmental assessment
   4. Respiratory and nutritional support
   5. Provide emotional and psychological support for patient and family

◆ XIII. Multiple sclerosis

A. Pathophysiology
   1. Results from progressive demyelination of the white matter of the brain and spinal cord
   2. Scattered demyelination lesions prevent normal nerve conduction
   3. After myelin is destroyed, neurologic tissue in the white matter of the CNS proliferates, forming hard yellow plaques of scar tissue; underlying axon fiber is damaged and nerve conduction is disrupted
   4. Possible causes
      a. Slow-acting viral infection
      b. Autoimmune response of the nervous system (autoantibodies produced against myelin)
      c. Allergic response
      d. Trauma
      e. Anoxia
      f. Toxins
      g. Nutritional deficiencies
      h. Vascular lesions
      i. Anoxeria nervosa

> **TEACHING TIPS**
> ## *Patient with multiple sclerosis*
>
> Be sure to include the following topics in your teaching plan for the patient with multiple sclerosis:
> 1. Perform an environmental assessment of the home to avoid or minimize risk of injury.
> 2. Participate in planned exercise program daily.
> 3. Avoid physical and psychological stressors whenever possible.
> 4. Eat a nutritious diet to maintain optimal body weight; reduce weight as needed.
> 5. Join a support group.

5. Precipitating factors include emotional stress, heat, overwork, fatigue, pregnancy, acute respiratory tract infection, and genetic (familial) factors
6. Remission may result from healing of demyelinated areas
7. More common in colder northern latitudes

B. Assessment
1. Signs and symptoms depend on location and extent of myelin destruction; extent of remyelination; and adequacy of subsequent restored synaptic transmission
2. Visual problems
3. Sensory impairment or paresthesia
4. Poorly articulated speech
5. Muscle weakness and spasticity
6. Hyperreflexia
7. Urinary and fecal problems
8. Intention tremor
9. Gait ataxia or dysmetria
10. Emotional lability
11. Sexual dysfunction
12. Fatigue

C. Interventions
1. Adequate rest and prevention of fatigue; good nutrition
2. Avoid precipitating factors when possible
3. Provide information from the National Multiple Sclerosis Society (for additional teaching tips, see *Patient with multiple sclerosis*)
4. Administer prescribed medications
   a. Corticotropin
   b. Corticosteroids
   c. Interferon-beta, Copolymer-1
   d. Imunosuppressants

      e. Antibiotics
      f. Antispasmodics
      g. Cholinergics
      h. Antidepressants
   5. Physical therapy
   6. Plasmapheresis
   7. Emotional support for the patient and family

POINTS TO REMEMBER

◆ The nervous system allows communication among different parts of the body and between the body and external environment.

◆ Synapses are one-way junctions across which electrical or chemical impulses are transferred from one neuron to another.

◆ The brain is the control center for most nervous system functions. The spinal cord primarily controls reflex responses.

◆ Nervous system disorders can affect the patient's body image, control over body functions, self-esteem, and fears of rejection, dependence, or dying.

◆ Nursing assessment for a patient who has a craniotomy should focus on changes in the LOC and on signs and symptoms of increasing ICP.

◆ Bacterial meningitis is the most common type of meningitis.

◆ Signs of meningeal irritation include nuchal rigidity and positive Brudzinski's and Kernig's signs.

STUDY QUESTIONS

To evaluate your understanding of this chapter, answer the following questions in the space provided; then compare your responses with the correct answers in appendix B, page 290.

1. Which two compensatory mechanisms protect the brain under adverse conditions? _____

2. When a patient has a seizure, which activities should the nurse observe and record? _____

3. What are the major causes of CVA?_____

_____

4. Which disorder is diagnosed with positive Brudzinski's and Kernig's signs?

_____

CRITICAL THINKING AND APPLICATION EXERCISES

1. Observe a lumbar puncture. Prepare an oral presentation for your fellow students describing the procedure and patient care.

2. Draw a diagram showing the physiology of increased intracranial pressure.

3. Interview a patient with a neurologic disorder. Evaluate the information for possible risk factors and identify ways to modify them.

4. Follow a patient with a CVA from admission through discharge. Develop a plan of care, including any need for follow-up and home care.

Musculoskeletal Disorders

CHAPTER OVERVIEW

The skeletal system, which consists of 206 bones, forms the framework that supports and protects the body. The muscular system animates the bones and JOINTS of the skeletal system. Together they are responsible for body movement. The health care professional must understand the structures and functions of the musculoskeletal system to comprehend the effects of musculoskeletal disorders in patients.

♦ I. Musculoskeletal system

A. Skeletal muscles
1. Attached to the bone
2. Muscle fibers arranged in long bands or strips (striations)
3. Voluntary: Unlike smooth muscle or cardiac muscle, skeletal muscles can be used at will

92

4. 600 known; classified according to location, action, size, shape, point of attachment, number of divisions, or orientation of fibers

B. Bone
   1. Classified by structure as cancellous or compact
   2. Classified by shape and location
      a. Long: such as arm and leg bones
      b. Short: such as wrist and ankle bones
      c. Flat: such as the shoulder blade
      d. Irregular: such as the jaw bone
      e. Sesamoid: such as the kneecap
      f. Axial skeleton: bones of the head and trunk
   3. Functions
      a. Protecting internal tissues and organs
      b. Stabilizing and supporting the body
      c. Providing a surface for muscle, ligament, and tendon attachment
      d. Moving, through lever action, when contracted
      e. Producing red blood cells, white blood cells (WBCs), and platelets in the bone marrow
      f. Storing mineral salts
   4. Bone formation and remodeling
      a. Bone-forming cells (OSTEOBLASTS) produce collagenous material (osteoid) which hardens upon mineralization
      b. Cells that break down bone (OSTEOCLASTS) reabsorb material from previously formed bones, allowing osteoblasts to build new bone
      c. Osteoblasts are mature bone cells in a resting state
      d. Longitudinal bone growth continues until adolescence; bone renewal continues throughout life, though it slows down with age
      e. Sex, race, and age influence bone characteristics
         (1) Bone mass
         (2) Bone's structural ability to withstand stress
         (3) Bone loss

C. CARTILAGE
   1. Nonvascular, noninnervated; supports connective tissue
      a. Made up of chondrocytes and various fibers
      b. Found mainly in joints, the thorax, the vertebral column and forms rigid yet flexible tubes (larynx, trachea, nose, ears)
      c. Temporary cartilage and cartilage of the fetal skeleton is replaced by bone
   2. Functions: supporting, cushioning, and shaping body structures
   3. Three types
      a. Hyaline: covers and protects articular bone surfaces
      b. Fibrous: forms the symphysis pubis and the intervertebral disks

     c. Elastic: located in the auditory canal, external ear, epiglottis, and the nose

D. Joints

    1. Union of two or more bones

    2. Three major types, classified according to how much movement they allow

      a. Synarthrosis: (no fluid present) permits little or no movement

      b. Amphiarthrosis: permits slight movement in all directions

      c. Diarthrosis: (some fluid present) permits free movement in any direction

    3. Also classified by shape and connective structure

      a. Fibrous

      b. Cartilaginous

      c. Synovial

E. BURSAE

    1. Small sacs of SYNOVIAL FLUID (viscous lubricating substance) in some diarthrotic joints, such as the knee and shoulder

    2. Located at friction points around joints and between tendons, ligaments, and bones

    3. Act as cushions, easing stress on adjacent structures

F. TENDONS

    1. Bands of fibrous connective tissue that attach muscles to the fibrous membrane that covers the bones

    2. Enable the bones to move when skeletal muscles contract

G. Ligaments

    1. Dense, strong, flexible bands of fibrous connective tissue that connect moveable bones of joints

    2. May either limit or facilitate movement

    3. Provide stability

♦ II. Movement

A. How it occurs

    1. Impulse from the nervous system and oxygen and nutrients from the blood stimulate the skeletal muscle

    2. Muscle contracts, applying force via the tendon to the bone

    3. Contraction force pulls one bone toward, away from, or around a second bone, depending on the type of muscle contraction and the type of joint involved

B. Types of movements

    1. Circumduction: circular motion

    2. Flexion: bending

    3. Extension: straightening

    4. Internal rotation: turning toward midline

5. External rotation: turning away from midline
6. Abduction: moving away from midline
7. Adduction: moving toward midline
8. Supination: turning upward
9. Pronation: turning downward
10. Eversion: turning outward
11. Inversion: turning inward
12. Retraction: moving backward
13. Protraction: moving forward

◆ III. Gout

A. Pathophysiology
   1. A metabolic disease marked by red, swollen, and acutely painful joints; found mostly in the foot, especially the great toe, ankle, and midfoot, but may affect any joint
   2. Hyperuricemia: urate concentration greater than 420 μmol/L; from overproduction of uric acid, underexcretion of uric acid, or both
   3. Primary gout
      a. Decreased excretion of uric acid
      b. Most likely cause: genetic defect in purine metabolism that causes overproduction of uric acid
      c. Predominantly occurs in men over age 30; occurs in 3% to 7% of postmenopausal women who use diuretics
   4. Secondary gout
      a. May develop secondary to another disease, such as obesity, diabetes mellitus, hypertension, leukemia, bone cancer, or kidney disease
      b. May be caused by certain drugs such as pyrazinamide
   5. Four stages of untreated gout
      a. Asymptomatic hyperuricemia: urate levels rise but patient is asymptomatic
      b. Acute gouty arthritis: painful swelling and tenderness
      c. Intercritical stage: patient may be asymptomatic or may experience exacerbation
      d. Chronic stage (tophaceous gout): tophi (clusters of urate crystals) may develop in synovial membranes, tendons, and soft tissue

B. Assessment
   1. Joint pain
   2. Redness and swelling in joints
   3. Tophi in great toe, ankle, and pinna of ear
   4. Malaise
   5. Tachycardia
   6. Elevated skin temperature
   7. Development of renal disorders

TEACHING TIPS
Patient with gout

Be sure to include the following topics in your teaching plan for the patient with gout:
• Avoid foods with high purine content, such as anchovies, broth, gravies, organ meats, mussels, sardines, scallops, or yeast.
• Avoid alcohol if taking colchicine or allopurinol.
• Avoid all aspirin-containing medicines; always check over-the-counter labels.
• Drink at least eight glasses of fluid per day.
• Avoid using an affected limb during acute episodes, especially if it is weight-bearing.

   C. Interventions

      1. Diet: low-purine, alkaline-ash; no shellfish, liver, sardines, anchovies, or kidneys; limit alcohol use

      2. Increase fluid intake to 3 L/day if not contraindicated

      3. Xanthine-oxidase inhibitors: allopurinol, probenecid, sulfinpyrazone (not for acute stage)

      4. Antigout agents: colchicine (in acute stage)

      5. Nonsteroidal anti-inflammatory drugs (NSAIDs)

      6. Intra-articular instillation of corticosteroids

      7. Provide information about the National Arthritis Foundation

      8. Reinforce exercise of joints

      9. For additional teaching tips, see *Patient with gout*

◆ IV. Osteoarthritis (degenerative joint disease)

   A. Pathophysiology

      1. Osteoarthritis occurs in diarthrodial joints and involves deterioration of the joint cartilage and formation of reactive new bone at the margins and subchondral areas of the joints; this deterioration results from damage to the cartilage cells (chondrocytes)

      2. Cartilage softens with age, narrowing the joint space

      3. Mechanical injury leads to thinning and erosion of articular cartilage

      4. Cartilage flakes enter the synovial lining, which becomes fibrotic, thus limiting joint movement; new bone called osteophyte (bone spur) forms at joint margins, also limiting movement (see *What happens in osteoarthritis*)

      5. Usually affects weight-bearing joints (such as knee, foot, hips, lumbar vertebrae)

   B. Assessment

      1. Pain relieved by resting joints and unrelieved by activity

      2. Joint stiffness; crepitus

What happens in osteoarthritis

The characteristic breakdown of articular cartilage is a gradual response to aging or to predisposing factors, such as joint abnormalities or traumatic injury.

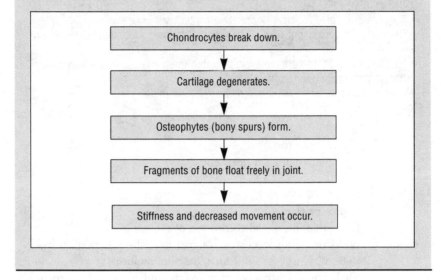

Chondrocytes break down.

↓

Cartilage degenerates.

↓

Osteophytes (bony spurs) form.

↓

Fragments of bone float freely in joint.

↓

Stiffness and decreased movement occur.

3. Heberden's nodules
4. Increased pain in damp, cold weather
5. Decreased range of motion
6. Joint enlargement

C. Interventions
1. Weight reduction
2. Balance of rest and exercise
3. For additional teaching tips, see *Patient with osteoarthritis,* page 98
4. NSAIDs or acetaminophen
5. Heat therapy
6. Cold therapy
7. Synovectomy, arthrodesis, joint replacement, arthroscopic lavage and debridement
8. Splinting; cane walker
9. Corticosteroid injections (short-term)

◆ **V. Osteoporosis**

A. Pathophysiology
1. Increased porosity of bone due to loss of bone mass
2. Bone mass is lost because of an imbalance between bone resorption and formation; resorption exceeds formation

---

TEACHING TIPS
Patient with osteoarthritis

Be sure to include the following topics in your teaching plan for the patient with osteoarthritis:
• Take analgesic medications prior to activities that precipitate pain.
• Find and follow a prescribed exercise program to maintain optimal range of motion.
• Maintain safety in the home to avoid falls (remove area rugs, install handrails in bathroom, maintain good lighting).
• Take a warm bath or shower upon rising in the morning.

---

   3. Predisposing factors
     a. Aging (changing sex hormone levels)
     b. Race
     c. Sedentary lifestyle
     d. Poor nutrition
     e. Decreased interstitial absorption of calcium
     f. Endocrine disorders (such as hyperthyroidism, hyperparathyroidism, Cushing's syndrome, diabetes mellitus)
     g. Medications (such as aluminum-containing antacids, corticosteroids, anticonvulsants)
     h. Cigarette smoking
     i. Excessive alcohol
     j. Positive family history
     k. Female gender

B. Assessment
   1. Pain
   2. Bone fractures
   3. Postmenopausal condition
   4. Thoracic kyphosis
   5. Gradual loss of height
   6. Decreased exercise tolerance

C. Interventions
   1. Prevention and early detection (see section V. part A. 3. Predisposing factors)
   2. Control bone loss, prevent fractures, and control pain
   3. Use of supportive devices such as a back brace
   4. Surgery, if indicated, to correct fractures
   5. Estrogen within 3 years after menopause to decrease the rate of bone resorption
   6. Analgesics and local heat to relieve pain
   7. Other medications
     a. Sodium chloride to stimulate bone formation

TEACHING TIPS
Patient with osteoporosis

Be sure to include the following topics in your teaching plan for the patient with osteoporosis:
• Develop and maintain a prescribed program of weight-bearing exercises.
• Maintain calcium intake at 1,500 mg/day (if postmenopausal).
• Maintain safety in the home to avoid falls (remove area rugs, install handrails in bathroom, maintain good lighting).
• Take vitamin D supplements unless living in a sunny climate.
• Discuss with the doctor the positive effects of medications, such as estrogen replacements or bone resorption inhibitors such as alendronate sodium.

  b. Calcium and vitamin D supplements
  c. Calcitonin to reduce bone resorption and slow the decline in bone mass
  d. Biophosphonates (such as etidronate) to increase bone density and restore lost bone
  e. Fluoride (such as alendronate) to stimulate bone formation
 8. A balanced diet rich in nutrients, such as vitamin D, calcium, and protein, that support skeletal metabolism
 9. For additional teaching tips, see *Patient with osteoporosis*
 10. Safety precautions include keeping side rails up on the patient's bed and moving the patient gently and carefully at all times; environmental assessment for safety hazards

◆ VI. Muscular dystrophy

A. Pathophysiology
 1. A group of congenital disorders characterized by progressive symmetrical wasting of skeletal muscles without neural or sensory defects
 2. Paradoxically, wasted muscles tend to enlarge because of connective tissue fat deposits, giving an erroneous impression of muscle strength (pseudohypertrophy)
 3. Caused by various genetic mechanisms
 4. Types of muscular dystrophy
  a. Two types (Duchenne's and Becker's) are X-linked recessive disorders, arising from defective gene coding for the muscle protein dystrophin; defect can be mapped genetically to the Xp21 locus
  b. Duchenne's (pseudohypertrophic) muscular dystrophy
   (1) Accounts for 50% of all cases
   (2) Strikes during early childhood and usually results in death by age 20
   (3) Mostly affects males, 13 to 33 per 100,000

    c. Becker's (benign pseudohypertrophic) muscular dystrophy
      (1) Occurs later in childhood or adolescence
      (2) Slower progression; patients usually live into their 40s
      (3) Mostly affects males, 1 to 3 per 100,000
    d. Facioscapulohumeral (Landouzy-Dejerine) muscular dystrophy
      (1) Slowly progressive
      (2) Involves muscles of face and shoulders
      (3) Usually does not shorten life expectancy
      (4) Autosomal dominant disorder
      (5) Affects both sexes about equally
    e. Limb-girdle muscular dystrophy
      (1) Involves muscles of pelvis, legs, and arms
      (2) Slowly progressive
      (3) Usually does not shorten life expectancy
      (4) Usually autosomal recessive disorder
      (5) Affects both sexes about equally

B. Assessment
  1. Duchenne's (pseudohypertrophic) muscular dystrophy
    a. Begins insidiously between ages 3 and 5
    b. Initially affects legs, pelvis, and shoulders
    c. Muscle weakness produces a waddling gait, toe walking, and lordosis
    d. Difficulty climbing stairs; falls down often
    e. Scapulae flare out when arms are raised
    f. Calf muscles become enlarged and firm
    g. Usually unable to walk by ages 9 to 12 and must use a wheelchair
    h. Weakening of cardiac and respiratory muscles leads to tachycardia, electrocardiogram abnormalities, and pulmonary complications
    i. Death commonly results from sudden heart failure, respiratory failure, or infection
  2. Becker's (benign pseudohypertrophic) muscular dystrophy
    a. Symptoms resemble those of Duchenne's (pseudohypertrophic) muscular dystrophy, but they progress more slowly
    b. Onset of symptoms around age 5
    c. Patients usually can walk well beyond age 15, sometimes into their 40s
  3. Facioscapulohumeral (Landouzy-Dejerine) muscular dystrophy
    a. Usually occurs by age 10 but develops during early adolescence
    b. Initially weakens the muscles of the face, shoulders, and upper arms
    c. Produces pendulous lip and absence of the nasolabial fold
    d. Inability to pucker mouth or whistle
  4. Limb-girdle muscular dystrophy
    a. Onset usually between ages 6 and 10

      b. Initial weakness in upper arms and pelvis

      c. Abdominal protrusion

  C. Interventions

    1. No treatment can stop the progressive muscle impairment

    2. Respiratory and cardiac support

    3. Refer patients for physical therapy

◆ VII. Septic (pyogenic) arthritis

  A. Pathophysiology

    1. Bacterial invasion of a joint, resulting in SYNOVITIS; spreads through the blood from a usually unknown primary site

    2. Effusion and pyogenesis can occur if organism enters the joint cavity

    3. Can lead to ankylosis and even fatal septicemia

    4. Most common organisms: *Staphylococcus aureus, Streptococcus pyogenes, Streptococcus viridans, Neisseria gonorrhoeae, Haemophilus influenzae, Escherichia coli, Salmonella,* and *Pseudomonas*

    5. Most common organism in children under age 2: *H. influenzae*

    6. Predisposing factors

      a. Any concurrent bacterial infection

      b. Serious chronic illness

      c. Alcoholism

      d. Old age

      e. I.V. drug use

      f. Autoimmune depression

      g. Articular or joint trauma

      h. Intra-articular injections

      i. Local joint abnormalities

  B. Assessment

    1. Severe joint pain

    2. Joint tenderness

    3. Local redness and edema

    4. Movement restriction

    5. High fever and chills

  C. Interventions

    1. Antibiotic therapy modified for specific organism

    2. Needle aspiration to remove purulent joint fluid

    3. Joint immobilization till movement can be tolerated

    4. Pain control; aspirin can cause a misleading reduction in swelling, hindering accurate monitoring of progress (see *Other types of arthritis,* page 102)

◆ VIII. Carpal tunnel syndrome

  A. Pathophysiology

    1. Chronic compression neuropathy of the median nerve at the wrist

Other types of arthritis

Intermittent hydrarthrosis—a rare, benign condition characterized by regular, recurrent joint effusions—most commonly affects the knee. The patient may have difficulty moving the affected joint but have no other arthritic symptoms. The cause of intermittent hydrarthrosis is unknown; onset is usually at or soon after puberty and may be linked to familial tendencies, allergies, or menstruation. No effective treatment exists.

Traumatic arthritis results from blunt, penetrating, or repeated trauma or from forced inappropriate motion of a joint or ligament. Clinical effects may include swelling, pain, tenderness, joint instability, and internal bleeding. Treatment includes analgesics, anti-inflammatories, application of cold followed by heat and, if needed, compression dressings, splinting, joint aspiration, casting, or possibly surgery.

Schönlein-Henoch purpura, a vasculitic syndrome, is marked by palpable purpura, abdominal pain, and arthralgia that most commonly affects the knees and ankles, producing swollen, warm, and tender joints without joint erosion or deformity. Renal involvement is also common. Most patients have microscopic hematuria and proteinuria 4 to 8 weeks after onset. Incidence is highest in children and young adults, usually occurring in the spring after a respiratory infection. Treatment may include corticosteroids.

Hemophilic arthrosis produces transient or permanent joint changes. Commonly precipitated by trauma, hemophilic arthrosis usually arises between ages 1 and 5 and tends to recur until about age 10. It usually affects only one joint at a time—most commonly the knee, elbow, or ankle—and tends to recur in the same joint. Initially, the patient may feel only mild discomfort; later, he may experience warmth, swelling, tenderness, and severe pain with adjacent muscle spasm that leads to flexion of the extremity.

Mild hemophilic arthrosis may cause only limited stiffness that subsides within a few days. In prolonged bleeding, however, symptoms may subside after weeks or months or not at all. Severe hemophilic arthrosis may be accompanied by fever and leukocytosis; severe, prolonged, or repeated bleeding may lead to chronic hemophilic joint disease.

Effective treatment includes I.V. infusion of the deficient clotting factor, bed rest with the affected extremity elevated, application of ice packs, analgesics, and joint aspiration. Physical therapy includes progressive range-of-motion and muscle-strengthening exercises to restore motion and to prevent contractures and muscle atrophy.

2. Median nerve supplies sensory innervation to the palmar surface of the thumb, the first two fingers, and part of the third; also supplies motor innervation for wrist and finger flexion

3. Compression of the median nerve in the space between the inelastic transverse carpal ligament and the bones of the wrist (carpal tunnel) leads to pain and numbness in the thumb, index, middle, and half of the ring finger

TEACHING TIPS
Patient with carpal tunnel syndrome

Be sure to include the following topics in your teaching plan for the patient with carpal tunnel syndrome:
• Decrease the amount of time spent on repetitive wrist movements (such as needlework, typing, or driving).
• Rest the wrist and hand as much as possible.
• Use a splint to immobilize the wrist and provide neutral extension.
• If symptoms persist, seek medical treatment.

4. The condition has numerous predisposing factors
   a. Strenuous, repetitive use of the hands
   b. Fractures and dislocations of the wrist
   c. Pregnancy, use of birth control pills, menopause
   d. Genetic
   e. Tenosynovitis
   f. Rheumatoid arthritis
   g. Acromegaly
   h. Hyperthyroidism
   i. Obesity
   j. Gout
   k. Amyloidosis
   l. Diabetes mellitus

B. Assessment
   1. Numbness, pain, paresthesia in the thumb and first two or three fingers; worsens at night
   2. Pain radiating to forearm, shoulder, neck, and chest
   3. Thenar atrophy (palm of the hand)
   4. Loss of fine motor movement of the hand

C. Interventions
   1. Surgical enlargement of carpal tunnel using endoscopy
   2. Limitation of fluids
   3. Elevation of hand
   4. For additional teaching tips, see *Patient with carpal tunnel syndrome*
   5. Use of hand splints
   6. Administration of analgesics, diuretics, glucocorticoids, NSAIDs
   7. Administration of vitamin B_6
   8. Avoiding manual activity that includes dorsiflexion and volar flexion of the wrist

POINTS TO REMEMBER

◆ Metabolic illnesses or medications that cause osteoporosis increase the risk of skeletal fracture.

◆ Alterations in mobility that result from a musculoskeletal disorder may affect a patient's development as well as economic, occupational, recreational, and social activities.

◆ Pain control is a primary focus for the nursing management of a patient with a musculoskeletal disorder.

STUDY QUESTIONS

To evaluate your understanding of this chapter, answer the following questions in the space provided; then compare your responses with the correct answers in appendix B, pages 290 and 291.

1. How are skeletal muscles classified? _____
   _____

2. When does the process of bone renewal stop? _____
   _____

3. Which pharmacologic agents are used to treat gout? _____
   _____

4. What characterizes osteoporosis? _____
   _____

CRITICAL THINKING AND APPLICATION EXERCISES

1. Observe an open-reduction internal fixation. Present an oral presentation for your fellow students describing the procedure and patient care.

2. Write a dietary plan for a patient with gout.

3. Interview a patient with a musculoskeletal disorder. Evaluate the information for possible risk factors and identify ways to modify them.

4. Follow a patient with a musculoskeletal disorder from admission through discharge. Develop a patient-specific plan of care, including any needs for follow-up and home care.

Infectious Disorders

LEARNING OBJECTIVES

After studying this chapter you should be able to:

♦ Describe the four types of infectious microorganisms and how they invade the body.

♦ Describe how the body naturally prevents infection.

♦ Recognize the signs and symptoms of septic shock.

♦ List three interventions for the common cold.

♦ Discuss the difference between the three major herpes infections.

CHAPTER OVERVIEW

An infection is a host organism's response to a PATHOGEN, or disease-causing organism. It results when tissue-destroying microorganisms enter and multiply in the body. Despite improved methods of treating and preventing infections — by means of potent antibiotics, complex immunizations, and modern sanitation — infection still accounts for much serious illness. Caring for a patient with an infection requires a sound understanding of the infection process. A thorough assessment is essential to planning and implementing appropriate care.

◆ I. Infectious microbes

A. VIRUSES
1. Primitive, microscopic parasites that may contain genetic material such as DEOXYRIBONUCLEIC ACID (DNA) or ribonucleic acid (RNA), but not both
2. No metabolic capability
3. Require living host cells to replicate

B. Bacteria
1. One-celled microorganisms that have no true organized nucleus and reproduce by asexual cell division
2. Pathogenic bacteria contain cell-damaging proteins that can cause cell injury and death
   a. Endotoxins: complex lipid and polysaccharide molecules released when the bacterial cell wall decomposes; can cause fever, bleeding, clotting, inflammation, and hypotension (endotoxic or septic shock)
   b. Exotoxins: proteins released by living bacterial cell during cell growth; enzymatically inhibit or modify key cellular elements leading to cell dysfunction or death

C. Fungi
1. Nonphotosynthetic microorganisms that can reproduce asexually (by cell division) or sexually
2. Larger than bacteria and contain a nuclei
3. Two major types
   a. Yeasts: round, single-celled, facultative anaerobes
   b. Molds: filamentous, multinucleated, aerobic microorganisms
4. Some fungi are part of the normal intestinal and oral flora; they become overabundant if the normal flora is compromised (such as when taking antibiotics)
5. Fungal infections are called mycotic because pathogenic fungi release mycotoxins

D. Parasites
1. Single-celled or multicelled organisms (protozoa, trypanosomes, helminths, arthropods)
2. Depend on a living host for food and protective environment
3. Uncommon except in hot, moist climates

◆ II. Barriers to infection

A. Defense mechanisms
1. Skin
2. Body secretions: most contain bactericidal substances, such as lysozymes and immunoglobulins; present in many organs
   a. Eyes

       b. Mouth and nasal passages

       c. Prostate gland

       d. Testes

       e. Stomach

       f. Vagina

       g. Bladder

   3. Ciliated cells

       a. Line the pulmonary airways

       b. Sweep foreign material from the breathing passages

   4. Mucus

       a. Viscous fluid secreted by specialized cells in GI and respiratory tracts

       b. Traps foreign particles and protects GI tract from digestive acids

B. Normal flora

   1. Harmless microorganisms that reside on and in the body

   2. Locations

       a. Skin: 100,000 microorganisms per square centimeter

       b. Nose

       c. Mouth

       d. Pharynx

       e. Colon

       f. Distal urethra

       g. Vagina

◆ III. Infection development

A. Opportunity

   1. Body's defense mechanisms break down

   2. Predisposing factors

       a. Humidity, other climate extremes

       b. Poor nutrition

       c. Stress

       d. Poor sanitation

       e. Crowded living conditions

       f. Pollution, dust, other airborne particulates

   3. Opportunistic infection: strikes people with altered, weak immune systems

B. Expansion

   1. Pathogen enters through several portals

       a. Direct contact

       b. Inhalation

       c. Ingestion

       d. Penetration as in insect or animal bites

   2. Pathogen attaches itself to a cell

       a. Releases enzymes that destroy the cell's membrane

b. Spreads through bloodstream and lymphatic system

c. Multiplies and causes infection in the target tissue or organ

◆ IV. Streptococcal infections

A. Pathophysiology

1. Small gram-positive bacteria, spherical to ovoid in shape and linked together in pairs of chains

2. Several species occur as part of normal human flora in the respiratory, GI, and genitourinary tracts

3. Species broken down into five classes: group A, B, C, D, and G

   a. Groups A, B, and D cause most infections

   b. Group A and B are hemolytic

   c. Most disorders associated with group D are caused by *Enterococcus faecalis* (formerly *Streptococcus faecalis* or *S. bovis*)

4. Three states of infection

   a. Carrier: infected but with no signs of infection

   b. Acute: tissues are invaded and cause physical symptoms

   c. Delayed nonsuppurative complications: specific complications associated with streptococcal infections occur

B. Assessment, diagnosis, and interventions (see *Comparing streptococcal infections*, pages 110 to 115)

◆ V. Salmonellosis

A. Pathophysiology

1. Caused by gram-negative bacilli of the genus *Salmonella*, members of the *Enterobacteriaceae* family

2. Most common species include *Salmonella typhi, S. enteritidis, S. choleraesuis,* and *S. typhimurium*

3. It occurs as gastroenteritis, bacteremia, localized infections, typhoid fever and, rarely, paratyphoid fever; results from contamination of food and water with feces of infected individual or asymptomatic typhoid carrier

4. Salmonella gastroenteritis is the most common infection in the United States, affecting 2 million people annually

5. Typhoid fever (*Salmonella typhimurium*)

   a. Uncommon in the United States

   b. Most severe form of salmonellosis

   c. Lasts 1 to 4 weeks

   d. Most patients are under age 30

   e. Most carriers are women over age 50

B. Assessment (see *Types of salmonellosis*)

C. Interventions

1. Antimicrobial therapy and antipyretics

(Text continues on page 114.)

Types of salmonellosis

TYPE	CAUSE	CLINICAL FEATURES
Bacteremia	Any *Salmonella* species, but most commonly *S. choleraesuis*. Incubation period varies.	Fever, chills, anorexia, weight loss (without GI symptoms), joint pain
Enterocolitis	Any species of nontyphoidal *Salmonella*, but usually *S. enteritidis*. Incubation period, 6 to 48 hours.	Mild to severe abdominal pain, diarrhea, sudden fever of up to 102° F (39° C), nausea, vomiting; usually self-limiting, but may progress to enteric fever (resembling typhoid), local abscesses (usually abdominal), dehydration, septicemia
Localized infections	Usually follows bacteremia caused by *Salmonella* species.	Site of localization determines symptoms; localized abscesses may cause osteomyelitis, endocarditis, bronchopneumonia, pyelonephritis, and arthritis.
Paratyphoid	*S. paratyphi* and *S. schottmuelleri* (formerly *S. paratyphi B*). Incubation period, 3 weeks or more.	Fever and transient diarrhea; generally resembles typhoid but less severe
Typhoid fever	*S. typhi* enters GI tract and invades the bloodstream via the lymphatics, setting up intracellular sites. During this phase, infection of biliary tract leads to intestinal seeding with millions of bacilli. Involved lymphoid tissues (especially Peyer's patches in ilium) enlarge, ulcerate, and necrose, resulting in hemorrhage. Incubation period, usually 1 to 2 weeks.	Symptoms of enterocolitis may develop within hours of ingestion of *S. typhi;* they usually subside before onset of typhoid fever symptoms. *1st week:* gradually increasing fever, anorexia, myalgia, malaise, headache, slow pulse *2nd week:* remittent fever up to 104° F (40° C) usually in the evening, chills, diaphoresis, weakness, delirium, increasing abdominal pain and distention, diarrhea or constipation, cough, moist crackles, tender abdomen with enlarged spleen, maculopapular rash (especially on abdomen) *3rd week:* persistent fever, increasing fatigue and weakness; usually subsides end of third week, although relapses may occur *Complications:* intestinal perforation or hemorrhage, abscesses, thrombophlebitis, cerebral thrombosis, pneumonia, osteomyelitis, myocarditis, acute circulatory failure, chronic carrier state

Comparing streptococcal infections

CAUSES AND INCIDENCE	SIGNS AND SYMPTOMS

STREPTOCOCCUS PYOGENES (group A streptococcus)

Streptococcal pharyngitis (strep throat)
• Accounts for 95% of all cases of bacterial pharyngitis
• Most common in children ages 5 to 10 from October to April
• Spread by direct person-to-person contact via droplets of saliva or nasal secretions
• Organism usually colonizes throats of persons with no symptoms; up to 20% of schoolchildren may be carriers. Pets may also be carriers.

• After 1- to 5-day incubation period: temperature of 101° to 104° F (38.3° to 40° C), sore throat with severe pain on swallowing, beefy red pharynx, tonsillar exudate, edematous tonsils and uvula, swollen glands along the jaw line, generalized malaise and weakness, anorexia, occasional abdominal discomfort
• Up to 40% of small children have symptoms too mild for diagnosis.
• Fever abates in 3 to 5 days; nearly all symptoms subside within a week.

Scarlet fever (scarlatina)
• Usually follows streptococcal pharyngitis; may follow wound infections or puerperal sepsis
• Caused by streptococcal strain that releases an erythrogenic toxin
• Most common in children ages 2 to 10
• Spread by inhalation or direct contact

• Streptococcal sore throat, fever, strawberry tongue, fine erythematous rash that blanches on pressure and resembles sunburn with goosebumps
• Rash usually appearing first on upper chest, then spreads to neck, abdomen, legs, and arms, sparing soles and palms; flushed cheeks, pallor around mouth
• Skin sheds during convalescence.

Erysipelas
Streptococcal gangrene (necrotizing fasciitis)
• Occurs primarily in infants and adults over age 30
• Usually follows strep throat
• Exact mode of spread to shin unknown

• Sudden onset, with reddened, swollen, raised lesions (skin looks like an orange peel), usually on face and scalp, bordered by areas that often contain easily ruptured blebs filled with yellow-tinged fluid. Lesions sting and itch. Lesions on the trunk, arms, or legs usually affect incision or wound sites.
• Other signs and symptoms: vomiting, fever, headache, cervical lymphadenopathy, sore throat

---

Impetigo (streptococcal pyoderma)
• Common in poor children ages 2 to 5 in hot, humid weather; high rate of familial spread
• Predisposing factors: close contact in schools, overcrowded living quarters, poor skin hygiene, minor skin trauma
• May spread by direct contact, environmental contamination, or arthropod vector

• Small macules rapidly develop into vesicles, then become pustular and encrusted, causing pain, surrounding erythema, regional adenitis, cellulitis, and itching. Scratching spreads infection.
• Lesions commonly affect the face, heal slowly, and leave depigmented areas.

DIAGNOSIS	COMPLICATIONS	TREATMENT AND SPECIAL CONSIDERATIONS
• Clinically indistinguishable from viral pharyngitis • Throat culture shows group A beta-hemolytic streptococci (carriers have positive throat culture). • Elevated white blood cell (WBC) count • Serology shows a fourfold rise in streptozyme titers during convalescence.	• Acute otitis media or acute sinusitis occurs most frequently. • Rarely, bacteremic spread may cause arthritis, endocarditis, meningitis, osteomyelitis, or liver abscess. • Poststreptococcal sequelae: acute rheumatic fever or acute glomerulonephritis • Reye's syndrome	• Penicillin or erythromycin, analgesics, and antipyretics • Stress the need for bed rest and isolation from other children for 24 hours after antibiotic therapy begins. Patient should finish prescription, even if signs and symptoms subside; abscess, glomerulonephritis, and rheumatic fever can occur. • Tell the patient not to skip doses and to properly dispose of soiled tissues.
• Characteristic rash and strawberry tongue • Culture and Gram stain show *S. pyogenes* from nasopharynx. • Granulocytosis	• Although rare, complications may include high fever, arthritis, jaundice, pneumonia, pericarditis, and peritonsillar abscess.	• Penicillin or erythromycin • Isolation for first 24 hours • Carefully dispose of purulent discharge. • Stress the need for prompt and complete antibiotic treatment.
• Typical reddened lesions • Culture taken from edge of lesions shows group A beta-hemolytic streptococci. • Throat culture is almost always positive for group A beta-hemolytic streptococci.	• Untreated lesions on trunk, arms, or legs may involve large body areas and lead to death.	• Penicillin or erythromycin I.V. or by mouth • Cold packs, analgesics (aspirin and codeine for local discomfort), topical anesthetics • Prevention: prompt treatment of streptococcal infections and drainage and secretion precautions
• Characteristic lesions with honey-colored crust • Culture and Gram stain of swabbed lesions show *S. pyogenes*.	• Septicemia (rare) • Ecthyma, a form of impetigo with deep ulcers	• Penicillin I.V. or by mouth, or erythromycin, or antibiotic ointments • Frequent washing of lesions with antiseptics, such as povidone-iodine or antibacterial soap, followed by thorough drying • Isolation of patient with draining wounds • Prevention: good hygiene and proper wound care

(continued)

Comparing streptococcal infections (continued)

CAUSES AND INCIDENCE	SIGNS AND SYMPTOMS
STREPTOCOCCUS PYOGENES (group A streptococcus) (continued)	
Streptococcal gangrene (necrotizing fasciitis) • More common in elderly patients with arteriosclerotic vascular disease or diabetes • Predisposing factors: surgery, wounds, skin ulcers, diabetes, peripheral vascular disease • Spread by direct contact	• Mimics gas gangrene; within 72 hours of onset, patient shows red-streaked, painful skin lesion with dusky red surrounding tissue. Bullae with yellow or reddish black fluid develop and rupture. • Other signs and symptoms: fever, tachycardia, lethargy, prostration, disorientation, hypotension, jaundice, hypovolemia, severe pain followed by anesthesia (due to nerve destruction)
STREPTOCOCCUS AGALACTIAE (group B streptococcus)	
Neonatal group B streptococcal infections • Incidence of early onset infection (age 5 days or less): 2/1,000 live births • Incidence of late-onset infection (ages 7 days to 3 months): 1/1,000 live births • Spread by vaginal delivery or hands of nursery staff • Predisposing factors: maternal genital tract colonization, membrane rupture over 24 hours before delivery, crowded nursery	• Early onset: bacteremia, pneumonia, and meningitis; mortality from 14% for infants over 1,500 g at birth to 61% for infants under 1,500 g at birth • Late onset: bacteremia with meningitis, fever, and bone and joint involvement; mortality 15% to 20% • Other signs and symptoms, such as skin lesions, depend on the site affected.
Adult group B streptococcal infections • Most adult infections occur in postpartum women, usually in the form of endometritis or wound infection following cesarean section. • Incidence of group B streptococcal endometritis: 1.3/1,000 live births	• Fever, malaise, uterine tenderness • Change in lochia
STREPTOCOCCUS PNEUMONIAE (group D streptococcus)	
Pneumococcal pneumonia • Accounts for 70% of all cases of bacterial pneumonia • More common in men, elderly, Blacks, and Native Americans, in winter and early spring • Spread by air and contact with infective secretions • Predisposing factors: trauma, viral infection, underlying pulmonary disease, overcrowded living quarters, chronic diseases, immunodeficiency • Among the 10 leading causes of death in the United States	• Sudden onset with severe shaking chills, temperature of 102° to 105° F (39° to 41° C), bacteremia, cough (with thick, scanty, blood-tinged sputum) accompanied by pleuritic pain • Malaise, weakness, and prostration common • Tachypnea, anorexia, nausea, and vomiting less common • Severity of pneumonia usually due to host's cellular defenses, not bacterial virulence

DIAGNOSIS	COMPLICATIONS	TREATMENT AND SPECIAL CONSIDERATIONS
• Culture and Gram stain usually show *S. pyogenes* from early bullous lesions and commonly from blood.	• Extensive necrotic sloughing • Bacteremia, metastatic abscesses, and death • Thrombophlebitis, when lower extremities are involved	• Immediate, wide, deep surgery of all necrotic tissues • High-dose penicillin I.V. • Good preoperative skin preparation; aseptic surgical and suturing technique
• Isolation of group B streptococcus from blood, cerebrospinal fluid (CSF), or skin • Chest X-ray shows massive infiltrate similar to that of respiratory distress syndrome or pneumonia.	• Overwhelming pneumonia, sepsis, and death • Bacteremia followed by meningitis or endocarditis	• Penicillin or ampicillin and an aminoglycoside I.V. • Patient isolation is unnecessary unless open draining lesion is present, but careful hand washing is essential. If draining lesion is present, take drainage and secretion precautions. • Vaccine in development
• Isolation of group B streptococcus from blood or infection site	• Bacteremia followed by meningitis or endocarditis	• Ampicillin or penicillin I.V. • Careful observation for symptoms of infection following delivery • Drainage and secretion precautions
• Gram stain of sputum shows gram-positive diplococci; culture shows *S. pneumoniae*. • Chest X-ray shows lobular consolidation in adults; bronchopneumonia in children and in the elderly • Elevated WBC count. • Blood cultures often positive for *S. pneumoniae*.	• Pleural effusion occurs in 25% of patients. • Pericarditis (rare) • Lung abscess (rare) • Bacteremia • Disseminated intravascular coagulation • Death possible if bacteremia is present	• Penicillin or erythromycin I.V. or I.M. • Monitor and support respirations, as needed. Record sputum color and amount. • Prevent dehydration. • Avoid sedatives and narcotics to preserve cough reflex. • Carefully dispose of all purulent drainage. (Respiratory isolation is unnecessary.) Advise high-risk patients to receive vaccine and to avoid infected persons.

(continued)

Comparing streptococcal infections (continued)

CAUSES AND INCIDENCE	SIGNS AND SYMPTOMS
STREPTOCOCCUS PNEUMONIAE (group D streptococcus) (continued)	
Otitis media • About 76% to 95% of all children have otitis media at least once. *S. pneumoniae* causes half of these cases.	• Ear pain, ear drainage, hearing loss, fever, lethargy, irritability • Other possible symptoms: vertigo, nystagmus, tinnitus
Meningitis • Can follow bacteremic pneumonia, mastoiditis, sinusitis, skull fracture, or endocarditis • Mortality (30% to 60%) highest in infants and in the elderly	• Fever, headache, nuchal rigidity, vomiting, photophobia, lethargy, coma, wide pulse pressure, bradycardia
Endocarditis • Group D streptococcus (enterococcus) causes 10% to 20% of all bacterial endocarditis. • Most common in elderly patients and in those who abuse I.V. substances • Often follows bacteremia from an obvious source, such as a wound infection or I.V. insertion site infection • Most cases are subacute.	• Weakness, fatigability, weight loss, fever, night sweats, anorexia, arthralgia, splenomegaly, new systolic murmur

2. Localized abscesses may need surgical drainage
3. Fluid and electrolyte replacement
4. All infections caused by *Salmonella* must be reported to the state department of health
5. Enteric precautions until three consecutive stool cultures are negative; the first one 48 hours after antibiotic treatment ends, two more at 24-hour intervals
6. Oral or parenteral typhoid vaccine
7. Cholecystectomy (carriers)

◆ **VI. Septic shock**

A. Pathophysiology
   1. Associated with massive systemic infection, which leads to release of numerous vasoactive substances, with widespread effects

DIAGNOSIS	COMPLICATIONS	TREATMENT AND SPECIAL CONSIDERATIONS
• Fluid in middle ear • Isolation of *S. pneumoniae* from aspirated fluid, if necessary	• Recurrent attacks may cause hearing loss.	• Amoxicillin or ampicillin and analgesics • Tell patient to report lack of response to therapy after 72 hours.
• Isolation of *S. pneumoniae* from CSF or blood culture • Increased CSF cell count and protein level; decreased CSF glucose level • Computed tomography scan of head • EEG	• Persistent hearing deficits, seizures, hemiparesis, or other nerve deficits • Encephalitis	• Penicillin I.V. or chloramphenicol • Monitor closely for neurologic changes. • Watch for symptoms of septic shock, such as acidosis and tissue hypoxia.
• Anemia, increased erythrocyte sedimentation rate and serum immunoglobulin level, and positive blood culture for group D streptococcus • Echocardiogram shows vegetation on valves.	• Embolization • Pulmonary infarction • Osteomyelitis	• Penicillin for *S. bovis* (non-enterococcal group D streptococcus) • Penicillin or ampicillin and an aminoglycoside for enterococcal group D streptococcus

    a. Massive vasodilation
    b. Hypotension
    c. Decreased venous return
    d. Decreased cardiac output (CO)
    e. Inadequate tissue perfusion
2. Occurs most among hospitalized patients
3. Approximately 25% of patients who develop gram-negative bacteremia go into shock
4. Two-thirds of septic shock cases result from gram-negative bacteria
    a. *Escherichia coli*
    b. *Klebsiella*
    c. *Enterobacter*
    d. *Proteus*
    e. *Pseudomonas*

    f. *Bacteroides*
5. Septic shock also results from gram-positive bacteria
    a. *Streptococcus pneumoniae*
    b. *S. pyogenes*
    c. *Actinomyces*
    d. *Staphylococcus aureus*
6. Other causative organisms
    a. Viruses
    b. *Rickettsia, Chlamydia*
    c. Protozoa
    d. Fungi
7. Predisposing factors
    a. Age: very young or very old
    b. Coexisting disease (such as malignancies, burns, acquired immunodeficiency syndrome [AIDS], diabetes mellitus, organ dysfunction)
    c. Poor nutrition
    d. Invasive devices
    e. Surgery
    f. Trauma
    g. Immunosuppressants

B. Assessment
1. Early stage (hyperdynamic; warm shock)
    a. Oliguria
    b. Sudden fever higher than 101° F (38.3° C)
    c. Chills
    d. Tachypnea
    e. Tachycardia
    f. Nausea or vomiting
    g. Diarrhea
    h. Prostration
    i. Vasodilation; warm, flushed skin
    j. Mental status changes
2. Late stage (hypodynamic; cold shock)
    a. Restlessness
    b. Apprehension
    c. Irritability
    d. Hypoglycemia
    e. Hypothermia
    f. Anuria
    g. Hypotension
    h. Altered level of consciousness (LOC)
    i. Hypoventilation
    j. Cold, clammy skin

C. Interventions
1. Identify and treat infection
2. Volume expansion
3. Respiratory support
4. Vasopressors
5. Temperature control
6. Treat acidosis
7. Nutritive support

♦ **VII. Lyme disease**

A. Pathophysiology
1. Caused by the spirochete *Borrelia burgdorferi,* carried by deer ticks
2. Tick injects spirochete-laden saliva into bloodstream or deposits fecal matter on the skin
3. After incubating 3 to 32 days, spirochetes migrate outward, causing a papular rash that becomes red and warm but is not painful (called erythema chronicum migrans)
4. Spirochetes disseminate to other skin sites or organs via the bloodstream or lymphatic system
5. Spirochetes may survive for years in joints or may die after triggering an inflammatory response in the host

B. Assessment
1. Three stages of Lyme disease
2. Stages overlap
   a. Stage 1 (acute stage)
      (1) Red lesion forms at site of tick bite
      (2) Lesion has a white center and bright red outer rim; it may itch, sting, or burn and usually disappears within 1 month
      (3) After several days, more lesions may erupt along with migratory, ringlike rash and conjunctivitis
      (4) In 3 to 4 weeks lesions fade to small red blotches, which last for several more weeks
      (5) The rash is commonly accompanied by fatigue, malaise, headache, fever, sore throat, stiff neck, nausea, muscle and joint pain, lymphadenopathy
      (6) Symptoms of palpitations and mild dyspnea reported in 10% of patients
      (7) Children may have fever as high as 104° F (40° C)
   b. Stage 2 (intermediate stage)
      (1) Some 60% of untreated patients develop asymmetrical joint pain, usually in the knees and hips
      (2) Erythema chronicum migrans may return weeks to months later if patients are not treated
      (3) Meningitis, cranial nerve palsies, and peripheral neuropathy

TEACHING TIPS
Patient with Lyme disease

Be sure to include the following topics in your teaching plan for the patient with Lyme disease:
• Avoid areas of dense foliage and high grasses.
• Wear clothing that completely covers arms and legs; tuck pants legs into socks or boots.
• Inspect skin and clothing for ticks after being outside.
• Use repellants rated safe for use on the skin. Reapply after bathing or swimming.
• Inspect pets frequently for ticks and remove the pests completely.

      (4) Less than 10% of patients in this intermediate stage have cardiac signs and symptoms
  c. Stage 3 (chronic stage)
      (1) Arthritis occurs 6 weeks to several years after initial tick bite in about 60% of cases
      (2) Usually only a few joints are affected, especially large ones
      (3) Recurrent attacks may lead to chronic arthritis with severe cartilage and bone erosion
      (4) May have chronic neurologic problems such as fluctuating meningoencephalitis with peripheral and cranial neuropathy

C. Interventions
  1. Prevention (for additional teaching tips, see *Patient with Lyme disease*)
  2. Adults: 14- to 18-day course of oral tetracycline, doxycycline, amoxicillin, or erythromycin
  3. Children: oral penicillin
  4. Later stage treatment may consist of I.V. or I.M. ceftriaxone
  5. Analgesics and antipyretics
  6. Corticosteroids and anti-inflammatories

◆ VIII. Common cold (acute coryza)

A. Pathophysiology
  1. About 90% of colds stem from viral infections of the upper respiratory passages and consequent mucous membrane inflammation
  2. Sometimes result from a mycoplasmal infection
  3. Incubation period from 1 to 5 days
  4. Over 100 viruses can cause the common cold
    a. Rhinoviruses
    b. Coronaviruses
    c. Myxoviruses

      d. Adenoviruses

      e. Coxsackieviruses

      f. Echoviruses

      g. Parainfluenza

      h. Respiratory syncytial virus

   5. Modes of transmission

      a. Respiratory droplets

      b. Contact with contaminated objects

      c. Hand-to-hand transmission

      d. See *What happens in the common cold,* page 120

B. Assessment

   1. During 1- to 5-day incubation period

      a. Pharyngitis, nasal congestion, coryza

      b. Headache, malaise, lethargy

      b. Burning and watery eyes

      c. Fever in children

      d. Chills

      e. Myalgia, arthralgia

      f. Nonproductive cough, nocturnal cough

   2. As cold progresses, feeling of fullness in head with a copious nasal discharge

   3. About 3 days after onset, major signs and symptoms diminish, but nasal congestion generally persists for about 1 week

   4. Colds are communicable for 2 to 3 days after onset of signs and symptoms

C. Interventions

   1. Aspirin or acetaminophen

   2. Rest

   3. Fluids

   4. Decongestants

   5. Vitamin C (controversial)

♦ IX. *Hantavirus* pulmonary syndrome

A. Pathophysiology

   1. New viral disease first reported in May 1993

      a. Distinctly different from the *Hantavirus* that causes disease in Asia and Europe (mainly hemorrhagic fever and renal disease)

      b. A member of the *Bunyaviridae* family, the *Hantavirus,* first isolated in 1977, is responsible for *Hantavirus* pulmonary syndrome

   2. Main mode of transmission is exposure to infected rodents, especially deer mice

What happens in the common cold

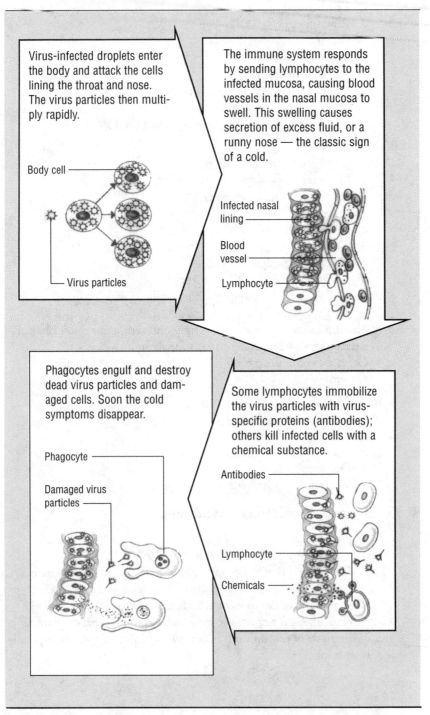

Virus-infected droplets enter the body and attack the cells lining the throat and nose. The virus particles then multiply rapidly.

Body cell

Virus particles

The immune system responds by sending lymphocytes to the infected mucosa, causing blood vessels in the nasal mucosa to swell. This swelling causes secretion of excess fluid, or a runny nose — the classic sign of a cold.

Infected nasal lining

Blood vessel

Lymphocyte

Phagocytes engulf and destroy dead virus particles and damaged cells. Soon the cold symptoms disappear.

Phagocyte

Damaged virus particles

Some lymphocytes immobilize the virus particles with virus-specific proteins (antibodies); others kill infected cells with a chemical substance.

Antibodies

Lymphocyte

Chemicals

    a. Infected rodents manifest no apparent illness but shed the virus in feces, urine, and saliva

    b. Human infection occurs through inhalation, ingestion of contaminated food or water, contact with rodent excrement, or rodent bites

    c. No evidence of transmission via mosquitoes or person-to-person contact

B. Assessment

  1. Prodromal period

    a. Fever, chills, myalgia, cough

    b. Headache, dizziness

    c. Nausea, vomiting, abdominal discomfort

    d. Adult respiratory distress syndrome

  2. Respiratory distress typically following onset of cough

    a. Hypoxia

    b. Hypotension, tachypnea, tachycardia

    c. Noncardiac pulmonary edema

    d. See *Screening for* Hantavirus *pulmonary syndrome,* page 122

C. Interventions

  1. Supportive treatment

    a. Adequate oxygenation; mechanical ventilation

    b. Stabilizing heart rate and blood pressure; fluid and electrolyte replacement

    c. Ribavirin in aerosol form may be useful

  2. Report all cases of *Hantavirus* pulmonary syndrome to the state department of health

  3. Prevention: Take precautions to reduce contact with rodents

◆ X. Rubella (German measles)

A. Pathophysiology

  1. Virus transmitted through contact with any of the following:

    a. Blood, urine, or stool

    b. Nasopharyngeal secretions; airborne transmission most common pathway

  2. Virus also crosses the placenta

  3. Incubation period 14 to 21 days; communicable from about 10 days before the rash appears until approximately 5 days after

  4. Strong teratogenic effect if mother exposed in the first trimester; fetus may have congenital cataracts, microencephaly, or deafness

B. Assessment

  1. Evidence from patient history

    a. Inadequate immunizations

    b. Exposure to someone with a recent rubella infection

Screening for Hantavirus pulmonary syndrome

The Centers for Disease Control and Prevention (CDC) has developed a screening procedure to track cases of *Hantavirus* pulmonary syndrome. The screening criteria identify potential and actual cases.

Potential cases

For a diagnosis of possible *Hantavirus* pulmonary syndrome, a patient must have one of the following:
• a febrile illness (temperature equal to or above 101° F [38.3° C]) occurring in a previously healthy person and characterized by unexplained adult respiratory distress syndrome
• bilateral interstitial pulmonary infiltrates that develop within 1 week of hospitalization with respiratory compromise that requires supplemental oxygen
• an unexplained respiratory illness resulting in death and autopsy findings demonstrating noncardiogenic pulmonary edema without an identifiable specific cause of death.

Exclusions

Of the patients who meet the criteria for potentially having *Hantavirus* pulmonary syndrome, the CDC excludes those who have any of the following:
• a predisposing underlying medical condition (for example, severe underlying pulmonary disease, solid tumors or hematologic cancers, congenital or acquired immunodeficiency disorders) or medical conditions or treatments — such as rheumatoid arthritis or organ transplantation — requiring immunosuppressant therapy (for example, steroids or cytotoxic chemotherapy)
• an acute illness that provides a likely explanation for the respiratory illness (for example, recent major trauma, burn, or surgery; recent seizures or history of aspiration; bacterial sepsis; another respiratory disorder such as respiratory syncytial virus in young children; influenza; or legionella pneumonia).

Confirmed cases

Cases of confirmed *Hantavirus* pulmonary syndrome must include the following:
• at least one serum or tissue specimen available for laboratory testing for evidence of *Hantavirus* infection
• in a patient with a compatible clinical illness, serologic evidence (presence of *Hantavirus*-specific immunoglobulin M or rising titers of immunoglobulin G), polymerase chain reaction for *Hantavirus* ribonucleic acid, or positive immunohistochemistry for *Hantavirus* antigen.

   c. Recent travel to an endemic area without reimmunization
2. Pinpoint maculopapular rash
   a. In many cases covers the face, trunk, and extremities within hours
   b. Small, red macules on the soft palate (Forschheimer spots) may precede or accompany the rash

c. By the 2nd day the rash begins to fade in reverse order in which it appeared; usually disappears by the 3rd day

d. Rapid appearance and disappearance of the rubella rash distinguishes it from rubeola (measles)

3. Low-grade fever (99° to 101° F [37.2° to 38.3° C]), usually disappears after the 1st day the rash appears

4. Palpation reveals suboccipital, postauricular, and postcervical lymph node enlargement as hallmark signs

5. Children usually do not have prodromal symptoms

6. Prodromal signs and symptoms in adolescents and adults
   a. Headache
   b. Malaise
   c. Anorexia
   d. Sore throat
   e. Cough

C. Interventions

1. Rash self-limiting, mildly pruritic; does not require topical or systemic medication

2. Antipyretics and analgesics for fever and joint pain

3. Bed rest unnecessary, but isolation precautions should be used until 5 days after the rash disappears

4. Only health care workers not at risk for rubella should provide patient care

5. Immunization with live rubella virus
   a. Should be given along with measles and mumps vaccines at age 15 months
   b. Repeat immunizations should be given to anyone immunized before 1960 and then every 10 years thereafter

6. Before immunizing anyone with the rubella vaccine, make sure they're not allergic to neomycin; pregnant; or immunocompromised and symptomatic

7. Advise women of childbearing age to avoid pregnancy by using an effective birth control method for at least 3 months after receiving the vaccine

8. For additional teaching tips, see *Patient with rubella,* page 124

9. Report confirmed cases of rubella to local public health officials

◆ XI. Herpes simplex

A. Pathophysiology

1. Herpesvirus hominis is a widespread infectious agent that causes both types of herpes simplex viruses (HSV1, HSV2)
   a. Type I: usually causes oral cold sores but can also cause genital herpes
      (1) Transmitted by oral and respiratory secretions

TEACHING TIPS
Patient with rubella

Be sure to include the following topics in your teaching plan for the patient with rubella:
• Stress the need to have children appropriately immunized.
• Pregnant women who have been exposed to rubella or who have never been immunized should receive counseling regarding the potential for birth abnormalities.
• Women who are pregnant or may be pregnant should avoid contact with individuals who have the disease.
• Do not receive active immunizations when respiratory or other infections are present.
• Encourage patients and families to maintain current record of immunizations.

      (2) Incubation period 2 to 12 days

   b. Type II: usually genital herpes but can also cause cold sores

      (1) Transmitted by sexual contact

      (2) Cross-infection may result from orogenital sex or autoinoculation

      (3) Incubation period 3 to 7 days

  2. Herpes simplex virus is a linear, double-stranded DNA molecule with an outer lipid-type membrane

  3. Mechanism of infection

   a. Virus binds to and enters cell cytoplasm

   b. Viral DNA is then injected into nucleus of host cell, causing it to manufacture more HSV particles, which are shed by the host cell

   c. Herpes simplex infection enters a latent state during which virus lays dormant in the dorsal root ganglia of sensory nerves supplying area involved

   d. Viral replication and redevelopment of herpetic lesions is called reactivation

B. Assessment

  1. Type I infection

   a. May cause generalized or localized infection as the virus invades the cells around the mouth

   b. Begins with fever and sore, red, swollen throat

   c. After brief prodromal period, primary lesions erupt

   d. Examination of the mouth may reveal edema and small vesicles (blisters) on a red base; these eventually rupture, leaving a painful ulcer followed by yellow crusting

   e. Vesicles commonly appear on the tongue, gingivae, cheeks, and lips

     f. Along with characteristic vesicles, the patient may develop sub-maxillary lymphadenopathy, increased salivation, halitosis, and anorexia

     g. Cervical lymphadenopathy

  2. Type II infection

     a. Tingling, burning, or itching in the area involved

     b. Malaise

     c. Dysuria

     d. Dyspareunia

     e. Leukorrhea

     f. Urine retention

     g. Localized, fluid-filled vesicles appear and may last for weeks

     h. In women, vesicles occur on cervix, labia, perianal skin, vulva, and vagina

     i. In men, vesicles occur on glans penis, foreskin, and penile shaft

     j. Lesions may also occur on the mouth and anus

     k. After vesicles rupture, they become shallow, painful ulcers with redness and edema, progressing to oozing yellow centers with crusting

     l. Inguinal lymphadenopathy may also be present

C. Interventions

  1. Medication to reduce pain and fever

  2. Anesthetic mouthwashes; cool compresses, sitz baths, and topical anesthetics

  3. Drying agents

  4. Petroleum-based salves or dressings can cause viral spread and slow healing

  5. Acyclovir is the drug of choice; valacyclovir and famciclovir also used

  6. Good hygiene

CLINICAL ALERT

◆ XII. Herpes zoster (shingles)

A. Pathophysiology

  1. Acute inflammation of the dorsal root ganglia of each spinal nerve

  2. Caused by herpesvirus varicella-zoster virus, same virus that causes chickenpox

  3. Vesicular skin lesions are usually confined to an area of skin supplied by branches from a single nerve

  4. Reactivation of the varicella-zoster virus causes shingles, but the trigger of the reactivation is unknown

     a. Virus may reactivate after lying dormant in the cerebral ganglia or ganglia of posterior nerve root

     b. Virus multiplies as it reactivates and antibodies from the initial chickenpox infection usually neutralize it

      c. If effective antibodies are absent, virus continues to multiply in the ganglia, destroying host neurons and spreading down the sensory nerves to the skin

B. Assessment

1. Pain within the dermatome supplied by sensory neurons of single or associated group of dorsal root ganglia
2. Fever
3. Malaise
4. After 2 to 4 days
   a. Severe, intermittent or continuous deep pain along affected dermatome(s)
   b. Pruritus
   c. Paresthesia
   d. Hyperesthesia in the trunk, arms, or legs
5. 48 to 72 hours after onset of pain
   a. Small, red vesicular skin lesions erupt and spread unilaterally around the thorax, trunk, face, and arms
   b. Skin lesions change into pus or fluid-filled vesicles, which may become infected
6. 10 to 21 days after rash appears, vesicles dry and form scabs
7. If trigeminal nerve is involved, lesions appear on the face, mouth, and eyes
8. If sensory branches of the facial nerve are involved, lesions appear in the ear canal and on the tongue

C. Interventions

1. Antipruritics, such as calamine lotion, or cool compresses
2. Analgesics such as aspirin, acetaminophen, or codeine
3. Systemic corticosteroid such as cortisone or corticotropin
4. Drug of choice is acyclovir (oral or I.V.), given to immunocompromised patients and those with infections of the ophthalmic branch of the trigeminal nerve; drug stops rash from spreading, reduces duration of viral shedding and acute pain, and prevents visceral complications
5. Valacyclovir and famciclovir may also be given
6. If other pain relief measures fail, treatment may include:
   a. Transcutaneous peripheral nerve stimulation
   b. Patient-controlled analgesia
   c. Nerve blocks
   d. Small doses of radiation
7. Ophthalmologic referral for eye involvement

◆ XIII. Infectious mononucleosis

A. Pathophysiology
 1. Caused by the Epstein-Barr virus, a member of the herpesvirus group
 2. Transmitted mostly via oropharyngeal route; called the "kissing disease"; may also be transmitted through sexual contact
 3. Approximately 80% of patients carry Epstein-Barr virus in the throat during the acute infection and for an indefinite period afterward
 4. Incubation period 4 to 8 weeks

B. Assessment
 1. Prodromal period
   a. Headache
   b. Malaise
   c. Profound fatigue
   d. Anorexia
   e. Myalgia
   f. Abdominal discomfort
   g. Chills
 2. 3 to 5 days after onset of symptoms
   a. Extremely sore throat
   b. Dysphagia
   c. Fever that usually peaks in the late afternoon or evening
   d. Lymphadenopathy
 3. Other possible effects
   a. Splenomegaly
   b. Hepatitis with hepatomegaly, nausea, vomiting, jaundice
   c. Stomatitis
   d. Exudative tonsillitis
   e. Pharyngitis

C. Interventions
 1. Treatment is mostly supportive
   a. Bed rest during the acute febrile periods
   b. Analgesics such as salicylates and nonsteroidal anti-infammatory drugs for headache and sore throat
   c. Warm saline throat gargles
 2. In cases of severe pharyngitis and airway obstruction steroids may be used

◆ XIV. Rabies (hydrophobia)

A. Pathophysiology

1. Acute central nervous system (CNS) infection caused by a virus that is transmitted by the saliva of an infected animal; occasionally, virus is transmitted via airborne droplets and infected tissue transplants

2. Almost always fatal if symptoms occur

3. Progression

    a. Virus begins to replicate in the striated muscle cells at the bite site

    b. Spreads up the nerve to the CNS and replicates in the brain, resulting in severe necrolyzing encephalitis

    c. Finally moves through the nerves into other tissues

B. Assessment

1. Presence of bite wound

2. After an incubation period of 1 to 3 months

    a. Local or radiating pain

    b. Sensation of cold, pruritus, tingling or burning at bite site

    c. Fever of 100° to 102° F (37.8° to 39° C)

    d. Malaise

    e. Headache

    f. Anorexia, nausea

    g. Sore throat

    h. Persistent loose cough

3. 2 to 10 days after prodromal signs and symptoms begin

    a. Hyperactivity

    b. Anxiety, apprehension

    c. Shallow respirations

    d. Altered LOC

    e. Ocular palsies, strabismus; asymmetrical pupillary dilation or constriction; absence of corneal reflexes

    f. Facial muscle weakness

    g. Hoarseness

    h. Temperature may rise to about 103° F (39.4° C)

4. Hydrophobia occurs in about 50% of patients

5. After about 3 days, progressive paralysis leads to coma and death

C. Interventions

1. Wound cleaning, debridement, and potential surgery; do not suture

2. Antimicrobial therapy for 3 to 5 days

3. Tetanus immunization

4. Rabies prophylaxis

    a. Risk assessment for rabies

    b. Confinement of animal for 10 days of observation

    c. Fluorescent rabies antibody, Negri bodies, and rabies antigen found in brain tissue of animal

    d. Passive immunization: human rabies immunoglobulin XI (rabies immune globulin); or equine antiserum (more likely to cause serum sickness)

    e. Active immunization: human diploid cell rabies vaccine (HDCV) or rabies vaccine adsorbed (RVA)

5. Preexposure prophylaxis for high-risk individuals (such as veterinarians and wildlife workers) with HDCV or RVA (still need prophylaxis if actually bitten)

6. Immunization of household pets

◆ XV. Ebola virus infection

A. Pathophysiology

1. Unclassified RNA virus; first appeared in Africa in 1976
2. Morphologically similar to Marburg virus
3. Four strains: Ebola Zaire, Ebola Sudan, Ebola Tai, and Ebola Reston
4. All four strains structurally similar but have different antigenic properties; Ebola Reston causes illness only in monkeys
5. Incubation period ranges from 2 to 21 days
6. Mortality up to 90%

B. Assessment

1. History usually reveals contact with an infected person
2. No clear line of infection may be apparent at the beginning of an Ebola virus outbreak
3. Flulike symptoms appear within the first 3 days of infection
4. As the virus spreads through the body inspection reveals bruising as capillaries rupture and dead blood cells infiltrate the skin
5. By 5th day of infection: maculopapular eruptions; black, tarry stools; hematemesis; epistaxis; bleeding gums
6. As infection progresses: dehydration, hemorrhage, liver and kidney dysfunction; in pregnant women, abortion and massive hemorrhage
7. At final stage: skin blisters and sloughs off; blood seeps from all body orifices; patient begins vomiting internal tissues; death usually ensues during 2nd week of illness from organ failure or hemorrhage

C. Interventions

1. No cure exists
2. Treat symptoms
3. Experimental treatment includes administration of plasma that contains Ebola virus–specific antibodies

♦ **XVI. Toxoplasmosis**

A. Pathophysiology

1. Caused by intracellular protozoan parasite *Toxoplasma gondii,* which affects both birds and mammals

2. Transmitted to humans through several routes

   a. Ingestion of tissue cysts in raw or undercooked pork
   b. Fecal-oral contamination from infected cats
   c. Blood transfusions
   d. Organ transplants
   e. Congenital (transplacental exposure)

3. Disease course

   a. Parasites emerge from ingested oocysts and quickly multiply within the GI tract
   b. Parasites (trophozoites) later spread to CNS, lymphatic tissue, skeletal muscle, myocardium, retina, and placenta; obligate intracellular organisms
   c. Cell death and focal necrosis occur, surrounded by an acute inflammatory response, the hallmarks of this infection
   d. Another form of the organism, the bradyzoite (cyst) contains viable trophozoites; once the cyst matures in the tissues, the inflammatory process becomes undetectable, and the cysts remain latent within the brain until they rupture.

4. In the normal host, immune response checks the infection, but in an immunocompromised or fetal host, focal destruction results in necrotizing encephalitis, pneumonia, myocarditis, and organ failure

5. Once infected, the patient may carry the organism for life

6. Reactivation of the acute infection may reoccur

B. Assessment

1. Over 80% of cases are asymptomatic

2. Mild, localized infection

   a. Malaise
   b. Myalgia, arthralgia
   c. Headache
   d. Fatigue
   e. Sore throat
   f. Fever
   g. Hepatosplenomegaly

3. Fulminating, generalized infection

   a. Headache
   b. Vomiting
   c. Cough, dyspnea
   d. Fever as high as 106° F (41.1° C)
   e. Delirium
   f. Seizures, focal neurologic deficits

      g. Maculopapular rash (except on palms, soles, and scalp)

   4. Congenital toxoplasmosis

      a. Hydrocephalus

      b. Microcephalus

      c. Seizures

      d. Jaundice

      e. Purpura

      f. Months or years later, strabismus, blindness, epilepsy, and mental retardation may occur

C. Interventions

   1. Most effective during acute stage

      a. Drug therapy with a sulfonamide and pyrimethamine for 4 to 6 weeks

      b. Folic acid to counteract the drugs' adverse effects, such as anemia and bone marrow toxicity

   2. Because drugs don't eliminate developed tissue cysts, patients with AIDS need toxoplasmosis treatment for life

   3. An AIDS patient who can't tolerate sulfonamides may receive clindamycin instead; this drug is also the primary treatment in ocular toxoplasmosis

   4. Report all cases of toxoplasmosis to the local public health department

POINTS TO REMEMBER

♦ A bull's eye-shaped rash signals the beginning of the Lyme disease syndrome.

♦ The rubella virus is communicable from about 10 days before the rash appears and until 5 days after.

♦ Initial infection of herpes simplex makes a carrier susceptible to recurrent infection.

♦ Rabies virus is transmitted from the bite of an infected animal and is almost always fatal once symptoms occur.

♦ Toxoplasmosis is transmitted to humans by ingestion of tissue cysts in raw or undercooked meat or by fecal-oral contamination from infected cats.

STUDY QUESTIONS

To evaluate your understanding of this chapter, answer the following questions in the space provided; then compare your responses with the correct answers in appendix B, page 291.

1. What type of infection is scarlet fever? _____

_____

_____

2. What are three common sources of salmonella transmission? _____

_____

_____

3. What are the early signs of Lyme disease? _____

_____

_____

4. What is a relatively new virus that is transmitted through infected rodents? _____

_____

_____

5. What differentiates rubella virus from rubeola? _____

_____

_____

CRITICAL THINKING AND APPLICATION EXERCISES

1. Observe some contaminated slides in the hospital laboratory. Compare and contrast the differences between organisms.

2. Develop a chart comparing different types of organisms.

3. Interview a patient with an infectious disorder. Evaluate the risk factors and identify ways to modify them.

4. Follow a patient with an infectious disorder from admission through discharge.

5. Develop a plan of care, including any needs for follow-up and home care.

Immune Disorders

CHAPTER OVERVIEW

The body protects itself from infectious organisms and other harmful invaders through an elaborate network of safeguards called the HOST DEFENSE SYSTEM or immune system. Caring for the patient with an immune disorder requires a sound understanding of the immune system. A thorough assessment is essential to planning and implementing appropriate patient care. Because the immunosuppressed patient is very susceptible to OPPORTUNISTIC INFECTIONS and further organ injury, all systems must be evaluated continuously.

♦ I. Host defense system

   A. Lines of defense
      1. Physical and chemical barriers
        a. Skin

      h, Mucous membranes
- 2. Acute inflammatory response occurs instantly, is nonspecific, and is of short duration
  - a. Major cells of inflammatory response are neutrophils and MACROPHAGES
  - b. Classic signs and symptoms of inflammatory response are redness, swelling, heat, and pain
- 3. Immune response is specific to an ANTIGEN and generates long-term memory for that antigen
  - a. T cells arise in stem cells and mature in the thymus
  - b. B cells arise in stem cells and mature in lymph nodes, spleen, and GI lymphoid tissues

B. Structures
- 1. Lymph nodes
  - a. Distributed along lymphatic vessels present throughout the body except for the brain
  - b. Filter lymphatic fluid that drains from body tissues and is later returned to the blood as plasma
  - c. Remove microorganisms and toxins from the circulatory system
- 2. Spleen
  - a. Largest lymphatic organ
  - b. Functions as a reservoir for blood
  - c. Contains macrophages that clear cellular debris and process hemoglobin
- 3. Tonsils
  - a. Made up of lymphoid tissues
  - b. Produce LYMPHOCYTES
  - c. Location in throat allows them to guard the body against airborne and ingested pathogens

◆ II. Types of immunity

A. Cell-mediated immunity
- 1. T cells respond directly to antigens
  - a. Destroy target cells (such as viruses or cancer cells) by secreting lymphokines
  - b. Probably originate from stem cells in the bone marrow; the thymus gland controls their maturation
- 2. Types of T cells
  - a. Killer cells: bind to the surface of the invading cells, disrupt the membrane, and destroy it by altering its internal environment
  - b. Helper (CD4+) cells: stimulate B cells to mature into plasma cells, which begin to synthesize and secrete IMMUNOGLOBULIN
  - c. Suppressor (CD8) cells: reduce the humoral response by B cells (see below)

B. Humoral immunity
1. B cells
   a. Responsible for humoral or immunoglobulin-mediated immunity
   b. Originate in the bone marrow and mature into plasma cells that produce ANTIBODIES
2. Types of immunoglobulin
   a. Immunoglobulin G (IgG): 80% of plasma antibodies; major antibacterial and antiviral antibody
   b. IgM: first immunoglobulin produced during an immune response; usually present only in the vascular system because of its large size, making it unable to cross membrane barriers
   c. IgA: found mainly in body secretions; defends against pathogens on the body surface, especially those that enter the respiratory and GI tracts
   d. IgD: present in plasma; easily broken down; predominant antibody on the surface of B cells; mainly an antigen receptor
   e. IgE: involved in immediate hypersensitivity reactions (allergic reactions); manifested within minutes of exposure to an antigen; stimulates the release of mast cell granules, which contain histamine, heparin, and other mediators
3. Complement system
   a. Major mediator of inflammatory response
   b. Consists of 20 proteins circulating as functionally inactive molecules
   c. Complement proteins cause inflammation by increasing vascular permeability, chemostasis, PHAGOCYTOSIS, and lysis of foreign cells
   d. Antigen-antibody reaction is usually needed to activate complement system

◆ III. Types of immune disorders

A. Immunodeficiency disorders
1. Result from an absent or depressed immune system
2. Examples: acquired immunodeficiency syndrome, severe combined immunodeficiency disease (AIDS), DiGeorge syndrome, chronic fatigue and immune dysfunction syndrome

B. Hypersensitivity disorders
1. Caused by an antigen entering the body
2. Reaction may be immediate or delayed
3. Types of hypersensitivity disorders
   a. Type I: IgE-mediated allergic reaction (antigen is called "ALLERGEN" in this type)
   b. Type II: cytotoxic reactions involving IgG and IgM antibodies

    c. Type III: immune complex reactions involving IgG and IgM antibodies

    d. Type IV: T-cell–mediated reactions

C. Autoimmune disorders

  1. The body launches an immunologic response against itself

  2. Autoimmune response leads to a sequence of tissue reactions and damage that may produce diffuse systemic symptoms

  3. Examples include rheumatoid arthritis, vasculitis, and systemic lupus erythematosus

◆ IV. Asthma

A. Pathophysiology

  1. A form of chronic obstructive pulmonary disease

  2. A chronic reactive airway disorder

  3. Airway obstruction results from bronchospasm, increased mucus production, mucosal edema, and fibrosis

  4. Two major forms of asthma: extrinsic (atopic) and intrinsic (nonatopic)

    a. Extrinsic asthma is associated with specific allergens: type I hypersensitivity

    b. Intrinsic asthma is a reaction to nonallergenic factors

  5. Course of extrinsic (atopic) asthma

    a. An allergen stimulates the production of IgE from B lymphocytes; IgE attaches to mast cells, causing degranulation and the release of histamine and other mediators

    b. Histamine attaches to receptor sites in the large bronchi, where it causes vasodilation, increased capillary permeability (smooth-muscle swelling), and bronchoconstriction—all causing decreased airway diameter

    c. *Slow-reacting substance of ANAPHYLAXIS* is a term for a group of vasoactive substances (histamine, prostaglandins, and leukotrienes) that are released during the inflammatory response and cause slow, prolonged vasodilation, increased capillary permeability, and constriction of smooth muscle in respiratory system

    d. Histamine also stimulates the mucous membranes to secrete excessive amounts of mucus, further narrowing the bronchial lumen

    e. On inhalation, the narrowed bronchial lumen can still expand slightly, allowing air to reach the alveoli; on exhalation, increased intrathoracic pressure collapses the bronchial lumen completely, resulting in air trapping and alveolar distention

    f. Mucus fills the lung bases, inhibiting alveolar ventilation; blood, shunted to alveoli in other lung parts, still cannot compensate for diminished ventilation

B. Assessment
  1. Mild asthma
     a. Patient has adequate air exchange and is asymptomatic between attacks
     b. Signs and symptoms include intermittent, brief (less than 1 hour) wheezing, coughing, or dyspnea once or twice a week
  2. Moderate asthma
     a. Normal or below normal air exchange
     b. Signs and symptoms include respiratory distress at rest, hyperpnea, or an abnormal increase in the depth and rate of respiration; exacerbations last several days
  3. Severe asthma
     a. Signs and symptoms occur continuously
     b. Signs and symptoms include marked respiratory distress, marked wheezing or distant or absent breath sounds, cough, paradoxical pulse greater than 10 mm Hg, chest wall contractions, tachycardia, apprehension, and restlessness

C. Interventions
  1. The best treatment is prevention, by avoiding precipitating factors such as allergens or irritants
  2. Desensitization to specific antigens, especially in children
  3. Medication
     a. Bronchodilators (such as theophylline, aminophylline, ipratropium, epinephrine, albuterol, metaproterenol, and terbutaline) decrease bronchoconstriction, reduce bronchial airway edema, and increase pulmonary ventilation
     b. Corticosteroids (such as beclomethasone, triamcinolone, hydrocortisone, and methylprednisolone) have the same effects as bronchodilators, as well as anti-inflammatory effects
     c. Mast cell stabilizers (such as cromolyn and nedocromil) are effective in patients with atopic asthma who have seasonal disease; prophylactically given to block the acute obstructive effects of antigen exposure by inhibiting the degranulation of mast cells
     d. Leukotreine modifiers (such as zafirlukast and zileuton) to decrease leukotriene-induced inflammation
  4. Oxygen
     a. Low-flow humidified oxygen to treat dyspnea, cyanosis, and hypoxemia
     b. Amount delivered should maintain the PaO_2 between 65 and 85 mm Hg
     c. Mechanical ventilation if no response to initial ventilatory support and drugs or patient develops respiratory failure

◆ V. Latex allergy

A. Pathophysiology

1. Latex is a substance that is found in an increasing number of products such as surgical gloves
2. Latex allergy is a type I or type IV hypersensitivity reaction to products that contain natural latex, derived from the sap of the rubber tree (*Hevea* species and others)
3. Allergy does *not* occur with synthetic latex products
4. The more frequent the exposure the higher the risk of an allergic reaction
5. Approximately 1% of the population has a latex allergy
6. 7% to 10% of health care workers are affected by latex allergy

B. Assessment

1. People who are frequently exposed to latex
2. History of asthma or other allergies, especially to bananas, avocados, tropical fruits, or chestnuts
3. History of multiple intra-abdominal or genitourinary surgeries
4. Frequent intermittent urinary catheterization
5. Urticaria
6. Flushing
7. Bronchospasm or laryngospasm
8. Pruritus
9. Palpitations
10. Abdominal pain
11. Swollen, teary eyes
12. Nausea
13. Diarrhea

C. Interventions

1. Best treatment is prevention: avoiding latex products
2. No allergy shots or cure for latex allergy
3. Allergic reactions treated with epinephrine, diphenhydramine, hydrocortisone

◆ VI. Anaphylaxis

A. Pathophysiology

1. An acute type I hypersensitivity allergic reaction
2. Causes sudden rapidly progressive cardiac and respiratory distress
3. Results from systemic exposure to sensitizing drugs or other antigens (such as penicillin, certain foods, iodine, insect venom, latex, animal sera)
4. Course of anaphylactic reaction
   a. Extreme type I hypersensitivity reaction; effects of mediators released by mast cells are systemic, not local (see section IV. Asthma)

    b. Systemic vasodilation can result in hypovolemic shock

    c. Capillary permeability changes lead to massive, generalized edema

    d. Severe bronchoconstriction

    e. Untreated anaphylaxis causes respiratory obstruction, systemic vascular collapse, and death (see *Understanding anaphylaxis*, page 140)

B. Assessment

    1. Anaphylactic reaction produces sudden physical distress within seconds or minutes but may be delayed up to 24 hours

    2. Initial signs and symptoms

        a. Feeling of impending doom or fear

        b. Weakness

        c. Sweating

        d. Sneezing

        e. Dyspnea

        f. Nasal pruritus

        g. Urticaria

    3. Cardiovascular signs

        a. Hypotension

        b. Shock

        c. Arrhythmias

    4. Respiratory signs and symptoms

        a. Nasal congestion

        b. Sudden sneezing attacks

        c. Profuse watery rhinorrhea

        d. Edema of upper respiratory tract (dyspnea, air hunger, wheezing)

    5. GI signs and symptoms

        a. Severe stomach cramps

        b. Nausea

        c. Diarrhea

    6. Neurologic signs and symptoms

        a. Dizziness

        b. Drowsiness

**CLINICAL
ALERT**

        c. Headache

        d. Restlessness

        e. Seizures

C. Interventions

    1. Prevention: avoidance of allergen

    2. Epinephrine

    3. Antihistamines (diphenhydramine)

    4. Corticosteroids

    5. Famotidine

    6. Oxygen therapy

Understanding anaphylaxis

The chart below outlines the sequence of events that occurs during anaphylaxis.

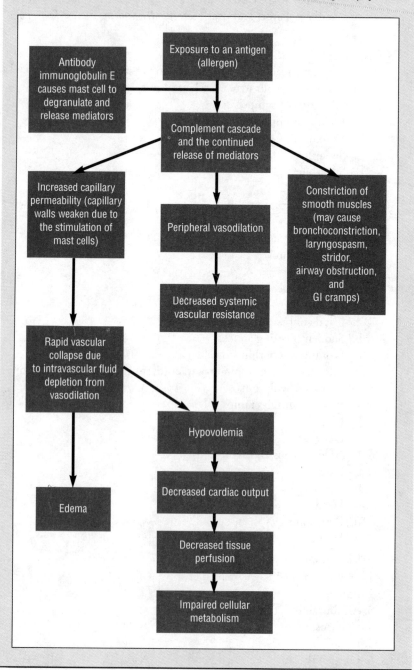

7. Medical identification bracelet

◆ VII. Rheumatoid arthritis

A. Pathophysiology
   1. A chronic, systemic, inflammatory immune disease; considered an autoimmune type III hypersensitivity disorder
   2. Attacks peripheral joints and surrounding muscles, tendons, ligaments, and blood vessels
   3. Spontaneous remissions and unpredictable exacerbations mark the course of this potentially crippling disease
   4. Cause is not known, but infections, genetics, and endocrine factors may play a part
   5. 70% to 80% of affected individuals have a substance called rheumatoid factor (RF), which is actually an antibody
      a. RF reacts with IgG to form immune complexes
      b. RF found in blood, synovial membrane, and synovial fluid
   6. Immune complexes in joint attract WBCs and macrophages; WBCs phagocytose complexes and release lysosomal enzymes in the process, leading to an inflammatory response
   7. Four inflammatory stages
      a. Synovitis develops from congestion and edema of the synovial membrane and joint capsule
      b. Pannus (a destructive vascular granulation tissue) covers and invades cartilage, eventually destroying the joint capsule and bone
      c. Fibrous invasion of the pannus and scar formation between joint margins; bone atrophy and misalignment cause visible deformities and restrict movement causing muscle atrophy
      d. Pain associated with movement may restrict active joint use and cause fibrous or bony ankylosis, soft-tissue contractures, and joint deformities
   8. Disease course characterized by exacerbations and remissions

B. Assessment
   1. At first the patient may complain of nonspecific systemic signs and symptoms (fatigue, anorexia, weight loss, and generalized aching and stiffness)
   2. As inflammation progresses through the four stages, specific symptoms develop, generally in the fingers; symptoms usually occur bilaterally and symmetrically and may extend to the wrists, elbows, knees, ankles, feet, and cervical spine
   3. Joint instability and limitation of movement
   4. Ulnar deviation of fingers
   5. Swan-neck or boutonniere deformity in hands
   6. Enlarged, misshapen joints
   7. Ankylosis

C. Interventions

1. Treatment aims to reduce pain and inflammation and preserve the patient's functional capacity and quality of life

2. Drugs

   a. Salicylates

   b. Nonsteroidal anti-inflammatory drugs (NSAIDs)

   c. Antimalarials

   d. Corticosteroids

   e. Disease-modifying antirheumatic drugs, such as gold salts, methotrexate, hydroxychloroquine, sulfasalazine, azathioprine

3. Therapeutic range-of-motion exercises

4. Surgery to reduce pain, realign joint surfaces, and redistribute stresses; joint replacements; arthrodesis

5. Joint rest (splinting)

6. Heat or cold therapy

7. Good posture and body mechanics

8. Assistive devices, such as canes and walkers

◆ VIII. Lupus erythematosus (LE)

A. Pathophysiology

1. A chronic, inflammatory, autoimmune disorder affecting the connective tissues

2. Two types

   a. Discoid lupus erythematosus

      (1) Affects only the skin

      (2) Superficial lesions; typically occur over the cheeks and bridge of the nose, leave scars after healing

   b. Systemic lupus erythematosus (SLE)

      (1) Affects multiple organs and can be fatal

      (2) Recurrent, seasonal remissions and exacerbations, especially during spring and summer

3. Exact cause of LE remains a mystery, but autoimmunity is probably the primary cause, along with environmental, hormonal, genetic, and possibly viral factors

4. In autoimmunity, the body produces antibodies against its own cells (autoantibodies)

   a. Resulting antigen-antibody complexes can suppress the body's normal immunity to bring on a chronic inflammatory response that causes tissue damage (type III hypersensitivity)

   b. Some complexes are antinuclear antibodies (ANA), others react directly with blood components and other antibodies (type II hypersensitivity)

5. The annual incidence in urban populations varies from 15 to 50 per 100,000 people

      6. SLE is 8 times more common in women than in men and is 15 times more common during childbearing years

      7. Occurs worldwide; more prevalent among African-Americans, Asians, and Hispanics than in Whites

B. Assessment

    1. Onset of SLE may be acute or insidious; no characteristic clinical pattern

    2. Patients may experience many signs and symptoms and have many concurrent conditions:

      a. Fever, anorexia, weight loss, malaise, fatigue, abdominal pain, nausea, vomiting, diarrhea, constipation, rashes, polyarthralgia, photosensitivity

      b. Blood disorders, such as anemia, leukopenia, lymphopenia, and thrombocytopenia, and elevated erythrocyte sedimentation rate (ESR) occur because of circulating antibodies

      c. Irregular menstruation or amenorrhea

      d. Joint pain that resembles rheumatoid arthritis found in 90% of patients

      e. Raynaud's phenomenon found in 20% of patients

      f. Cardiopulmonary signs and symptoms found in 50% of patients

        (1) Chest pain, indicating pleuritis, pleural effusion, pericarditis, pericardial effusion

        (2) Dyspnea

        (3) Tachycardia

        (4) Central cyanosis

        (5) Hypotension

      g. Neurologic effects

        (1) Seizure disorders and mental dysfunction may indicate neurologic damage

        (2) Emotional lability

        (3) Psychosis

        (4) Headaches

        (5) Irritability

        (6) Depression

      h. Urinary tract infections and renal failure are the leading cause of death for SLE patients

      i. Skin effects: rash on areas exposed to light—varying in severity from red areas to disc-shaped plaques; characteristic butterfly rash on nose and cheeks; patchy alopecia is also common in SLE

C. Interventions

    1. NSAIDs for arthritis and arthralgia

    2. Skin lesions require sun protection and topical corticosteroid creams, such as triamcinolone or hydrocortisone

    3. Fluorinated steroids may control acute or discoid lesions

4 Stubborn lesions may respond to intralesional or systemic cortico-steroids or antimalarials (hydroxychloroquine, chloroquine, dapsone)

5. Because hydroxychloroquine and chloroquine can cause retinal damage, patients receiving them should have ophthalmologic examinations every 6 months.

6. Corticosteroids are given for systemic symptoms, acute generalized exacerbations, and injury to vital organs; once symptoms are under control, dosage is gradually reduced and then discontinued

7. Cytotoxic drugs, such as azathioprine or methotrexate, to delay or prevent renal deterioration in some patients

8. Warfarin to prevent clotting in vascular structures

◆ IX. Scleroderma (systemic sclerosis)

A. Pathophysiology

1. A diffuse connective tissue disease of unknown cause characterized by fibrotic, degenerative, and sometimes inflammatory changes in the skin, blood vessels, synovial membranes, skeletal muscles, and internal organs; marked vasculitis and fibrosis

2. Affects more women than men, especially between ages 30 to 50; more common in blacks

3. Several distinctive forms

   a. CREST syndrome: benign form (characterized by *C*alcinosis, *R*aynaud's phenomenon, *E*sophageal dysfunction, *S*clerodactyly, and *T*elangiectasia)

   b. Diffuse systemic sclerosis: generalized skin thickening and invasion of internal organ systems

   c. Localized scleroderma: patchy skin changes with a droplike appearance known as morphea

   d. Linear scleroderma: marked by a band of thickened skin on the face or extremities that severely damages underlying tissues, causing atrophy and deformity; most common in childhood

   e. Other forms include chemically induced localized scleroderma; eosinophilic myalgia syndrome; toxic oil syndrome; and graft-versus-host disease

B. Assessment

1. Scleroderma begins with Raynaud's phenomenon—blanching, cyanosis, and erythema of the fingers and toes in response to stress or extreme cold

2. Raynaud's phenomenon may precede scleroderma by months or years

3. Later signs and symptoms

   a. Pain, stiffness, and swelling of fingers and joints

   b. Skin thickening, with taut, shiny skin over the entire hand and forearm

    c. Facial skin becomes tight and inelastic

    d. Gastroesophageal reflux, dysphagia, and bloating after meals

    e. Abdominal distention, diarrhea, constipation, malodorous floating stools, signs of malabsorption

  4. Advanced disease

    a. Cardiac and pulmonary fibrosis produce arrhythmias and respiratory failure

    b. Renal failure usually accompanied by malignant hypertension, the main cause of death

C. Interventions

  1. Currently no cure exists for scleroderma

  2. Treatment aims to preserve normal body functions and minimize complications, with organ or system-specific drugs such as penicillamine, physical therapy, and nutritional support

◆ X. Acquired immunodeficiency syndrome

A. Pathophysiology

  1. Causes progressive impairment of the immune response and gradual destruction of immune cells, including T cells

  2. Immunodeficiency renders the patient susceptible to opportunistic infections and unusual cancers

  3. Caused by infection of selected body cells with the human immunodeficiency virus (HIV), a retrovirus

  4. Average time between HIV exposure to onset of symptoms is 4.5 years

  5. Virus destroys $CD4^+$ cells (helper T cells), which regulate the normal immune response

  6. Modes of transmission

    a. Contact with infected blood or blood products

    b. Contact with infected body fluids

    c. Transplacental, from infected mother to the fetus

    d. Breast milk

  7. Classification of AIDS (Centers for Disease Control and Prevention [CDC] 1993)

    a. Clinical categories

      (1) Category A: persistent, generalized lymph node enlargement; acute (primary) HIV infection with accompanying illness, or history of acute HIV infection; may be asymptomatic

      (2) Category B: bacillary angiomatosis; oropharyngeal or persistent vulvovaginal candidiasis; fever or diarrhea lasting over 1 month; idiopathic thrombocytopenic purpura; pelvic inflammatory disease (especially with tubo-ovarian abscess); and peripheral neuropathy

(Text continues on page 148.)

Types of vasculitis

TYPE	VESSELS INVOLVED
Polyarteritis nodosa	Small to medium arteries throughout body. Lesions tend to be segmental, occur at bifurcations and branchings of arteries, and spread distally to arterioles. In severe cases, lesions circumferentially involve adjacent veins.
Allergic angiitis and granulomatosis (Churg-Strauss syndrome)	Small to medium arteries (including arterioles, capillaries, and venules), mainly of the lungs but also other organs
Polyangiitis overlap syndrome	Small to medium arteries (including arterioles, capillaries, and venules) of the lungs and other organs
Wegener's granulomatosis	Small to medium vessels of the respiratory tract and kidney
Temporal arteritis	Medium to large arteries, most commonly branches of the carotid artery
Takayasu's arteritis (aortic arch syndrome)	Medium to large arteries, particularly the aortic arch and its branches and, possibly, the pulmonary artery
Hypersensitivity vasculitis	Small vessels, especially of the skin
Mucocutaneous lymph node syndrome (Kawasaki disease)	Small to medium vessels, primarily of the lymph nodes; may progress to involve coronary arteries
Behçet's disease	Small vessels, primarily of the mouth and genitalia but also of the eyes, skin, joints, GI tract, and central nervous system

SIGNS AND SYMPTOMS	DIAGNOSIS
Hypertension, abdominal pain, myalgias, headache, joint pain, weakness	History of symptoms; elevated erythrocyte sedimentation rate (ESR); leukocytosis; anemia; thrombocytosis; depressed C3 complement; rheumatoid factor more than 1:60; circulating immune complexes; tissue biopsy showing necrotizing vasculitis
Resembles polyarteritis nodosa with hallmark of severe pulmonary involvement	History of asthma; eosinophilia; tissue biopsy showing granulomatous inflammation with eosinophilic infiltration
Combines symptoms of polyarteritis nodosa and allergic angiitis and granulomatosis	Possible history of allergy; eosinophilia; tissue biopsy showing granulomatous inflammation with eosinophilic infiltration
Fever, pulmonary congestion, cough, malaise, anorexia, weight loss, mild to severe hematuria	Tissue biopsy showing necrotizing vasculitis with granulomatous inflammation; leukocytosis; elevated ESR and immunoglobulin A (IgA) and IgG levels; low rheumatoid factor titer; circulating immune complexes; antineutrophil cytoplasmic antibody in more than 90% of patients
Fever, myalgia, jaw claudication, visual changes, headache (associated with polymyalgia rheumatica syndrome)	Decreased hemoglobin level; elevated ESR; tissue biopsy showing panarteritis with infiltration of mononuclear cells, giant cells within vessel wall, fragmentation of internal elastic lamina, and proliferation of intima
Malaise, pallor, nausea, night sweats, arthralgias, anorexia, weight loss, pain or paresthesia distal to affected area, bruits, loss of distal pulses, syncope and, if carotid artery is involved, diplopia and transient blindness. May progress to heart failure or cerebrovascular accident.	Decreased hemoglobin level; leukocytosis; positive lupus erythematosus cell preparation and elevated ESR; arteriography showing calcification and obstruction of affected vessels; tissue biopsy showing inflammation of adventitia and intima of vessels, and thickening of vessel walls
Palpable purpura, papules, nodules, vesicles, bullae, ulcers, or chronic or recurrent urticaria	History of exposure to antigen, such as a microorganism or drug; tissue biopsy showing leukocytoclastic angiitis, usually in postcapillary venules, with infiltration of polymorphonuclear leukocytes, fibrinoid necrosis, and extravasation of erythrocytes
Fever; nonsuppurative cervical adenitis; edema; congested conjunctivae; erythema of oral cavity, lips, and palms; and desquamation of fingertips. May progress to arthritis, myocarditis, pericarditis, myocardial infarction, and cardiomegaly.	History of symptoms; elevated ESR; tissue biopsy showing intimal proliferation and infiltration of vessel walls with mononuclear cells; echocardiography necessary
Recurrent oral ulcers, eye lesions, genital lesions, and cutaneous lesions	History of symptoms

(3) Category C: candidiasis of the bronchi, trachea, lungs, or esophagus; invasive cervical cancer; disseminated or extrapulmonary coccidiomycosis; extrapulmonary cryptococcosis; chronic intestinal cryptosporidiosis; cytomegalovirus (CMV) disease affecting organs other than the liver, spleen, or lymph nodes; CMV retinitis with vision loss; encephalopathy related to HIV; herpes simplex involving chronic ulcers or hepatic bronchitis, pneumonitis or esophagitis; disseminated or extrapulmonary histoplasmosis; chronic intestinal isosporiasis; Kaposi's sarcoma; Burkitt's lymphoma or its equivalent; immunoblastic lymphoma or its equivalent; primary brain lymphoma; disseminated or extrapulmonary *Mycobacterium avium* complex or *M. kansasii*; disseminated or extrapulmonary *M. tuberculosis*; any other species of *Mycobacterium* (disseminated or extrapulmonary); *Pneumocystis carinii* pneumonia; recurrent pneumonia; progressive multifocal leukoencephalopathy; recurrent *Salmonella* septicemia; toxoplasmosis of the brain; wasting syndrome caused by HIV

   b. CD4+ (helper T-cell) count categories
     (1) ≥ 500 µg/L
     (2) 200 to 499 µg/L
     (3) < 200 µg/L (AIDS indicator T-cell count)

B. Assessment
  1. Patient may have no symptoms for years after exposure
  2. Neurologic symptoms from HIV encephalopathy
  3. Symptoms of an opportunistic infection
  4. Symptoms of Kaposi's sarcoma, lymphomas

C. Interventions
  1. No cure exists at the present time
  2. Administer prescribed medications
    a. Antiretrovirals
    b. Immunomodulators
    c. Anti-infectives
    d. Analgesics
    e. Protease or reverse transcriptase inhibitors
    f. Combinations of drugs ("AIDS cocktails")
  3. Treat specific opportunistic infections, organ system dysfunction, or both
  4. Maintain standard precautions
  5. Provide psychosocial, financial, or occupational support

◆ XI. Vasculitis

A. Pathophysiology

1. Broad spectrum of disorders characterized by inflammation and necrosis of blood vessels
2. Clinical effects depend on the vessels involved and reflect tissue ischemia caused by blood flow obstruction
3. Prognosis is variable
4. May be a primary disorder or occur secondary to other disorders
5. One theory of disease development
   a. Initiated by excessive circulating antigen, which triggers the formation of soluble antigen-antibody complexes
   b. Complexes cannot be effectively cleared by the reticuloendothelial system and are deposited in the blood vessels
   c. The deposited complexes activate the complement cascade, resulting in chemotaxis of neutrophils, which release lysosomal enzymes
   d. Lysosomal enzymes cause vessel damage and necrosis, which may precipitate thrombosis, occlusion, hemorrhage, and ischemia
6. Another theory
   a. Circulating antigen triggers the release of soluble mediators by sensitized lymphocytes, which attract macrophages
   b. Macrophages release intracellular enzymes, which cause vascular damage
   c. Macrophages can also transform into epithelioid and multinucleated giant cells that typify the granulomatous vasculitides
   d. Phagocytosis of immune complexes by macrophages enhances granuloma formation

B. Assessment
1. Clinical effects depend on vessels involved
2. See *Types of vasculitis,* pages 146 and 147, for signs and symptoms and diagnostic measures

C. Interventions
1. Remove offending antigen
2. Administer prescribed medications
   a. Anti-inflammatory agents
   b. Immunosuppressants
   c. Cytotoxins
   d. Analgesics
3. Treat underlying disorder (in secondary vasculitis)
4. Provide emotional support to patient and family

POINTS TO REMEMBER

♦ In autoimmunity, the body produces antibodies against its own cells.

◆ Anaphylaxis is always an emergency.

◆ Rheumatoid arthritis usually requires lifelong treatment and sometimes surgery.

◆ The CDC recommends testing for HIV be done immediately after and 3 months after exposure. Antibodies can be detected 3 to 27 weeks after infection.

STUDY QUESTIONS

To evaluate your understanding of this chapter, answer the following questions in the space provided; then compare your responses with the correct answers in appendix B, page 291.

1. Which immunoglobulin is responsible for immediate hypersensitivity reactions? _____

_____

2. What are three common complaints associated with rheumatoid arthritis?

_____

_____

3. What signs and symptoms characterize lupus erythematosus?_____

_____

_____

4. What are the four modes of transmission of HIV? _____

_____

CRITICAL THINKING AND APPLICATION EXERCISES

1. Interview a patient with an immune disorder. Evaluate the information for possible risk factors and identify ways to modify them.

2. Follow a patient with an immune disorder from admission to discharge. Develop a plan of care, including any need for follow-up or home care.

3. Observe an arthroscopy. Prepare an oral report for your fellow students describing the procedure and the appropriate patient care.

Gastrointestinal Disorders

LEARNING OBJECTIVES

After studying this chapter you should be able to:

♦ Describe the structures and functions of the digestive system and related organs.

♦ Differentiate between modifiable and nonmodifiable risk factors in the development of a GI disorder.

♦ List three probable and three possible nursing diagnoses for a patient with a GI disorder.

♦ Identify the nursing interventions for a patient with a GI disorder.

CHAPTER OVERVIEW

The GI system is the body's food processing complex. It performs the critical task of supplying essential nutrients to fuel the other organs and body systems. A malfunction along the GI tract or in one of the accessory glands or organs can produce far-reaching metabolic effects, which may become life-threatening. Caring for the patient with a GI disorder requires a sound understanding of GI anatomy, physiology, and function. A thorough assessment is essential to planning and implementing appropriate patient care.

♦ **I. GI tract**

    A. Structures
       1. Mouth
       2. Esophagus

3. Stomach
4. Small intestine
5. Large intestine

B. Function
1. Mouth: chewing and salivation softens food, making it easy to swallow
   a. Ptyalin, an enzyme in saliva, begins to convert starches to sugars
   b. After swallowing, the upper esophageal sphincter relaxes, allowing chewed food to enter the esophagus
2. Esophagus: peristaltic waves activated by the glossopharyngeal nerve propel food toward the stomach
3. Stomach: As food enters the stomach, stomach wall distends
   a. Mucosal lining releases gastrin, which stimulates hydrochloric ACID secretion and stimulates stomach's motor function, or peristalsis
   b. Three major motor functions of stomach: holding food, mixing food with gastric juices (chyme), and slowly parceling chyme into the small intestine for further DIGESTION and absorption
4. Small intestine: approximately 20' (6.1 m) long; locus of nearly all nutrient absorption; four major parts
   a. Pylorus: narrow opening between the stomach and the duodenum
   b. Duodenum: C-shaped curve that extends from the stomach to the jejunum
   c. Oddi's sphincter: opening in the duodenum through which bile and pancreatic enzymes enter the intestine to neutralize the acidic chyme and aid digestion
   d. Jejunum: extends from the duodenum and forms the longest portion of the small intestine; leads to the ileum
5. Large intestine: locus of water absorption (except for about 100 ml)
   a. Ileocecal valve located at end of small intestine; a sphincter that empties nutrient-depleted chyme into the large intestine
   b. Chyme, consisting of mostly indigestible material, enters the ascending colon at the cecum, an outpouching at beginning of the large intestine
   c. Chyme passes through the transverse colon, the descending colon, and finally to the rectum and anal canal, where it is expelled

◆ II. Stomatitis

A. Pathophysiology
1. A common infection; inflammation of the oral mucosa, which may also extend to the buccal mucosa, lips, and palate
2. Two main types

    a. Acute herpetic stomatitis
      (1) Results from herpes simplex virus
      (2) Characterized by vesicular eruption on mucous membranes of mouth and pharynx
      (3) Usually self-limiting; however, it may be severe and in newborns may be generalized and potentially fatal
      (4) Common in children ages 1 to 3
    b. Aphthous stomatitis
      (1) Cause unknown
      (2) Predisposing factors include stress, fatigue, anxiety, febrile states, trauma, and overexposure to the sun
      (3) Common in girls and female adolescents
      (4) Usually heals spontaneously without scarring in 10 to 14 days
    c. Other oral infections include gingivitis, periodontitis, Vincent's angina, and glossitis (see *Types of oral infections,* page 154)

B. Assessment
  1. Acute herpetic stomatitis
    a. Sudden onset of mouth pain, malaise, lethargy, anorexia, irritability, and fever, which may last for 1 to 2 weeks
    b. Gums are swollen and bleed easily
    c. Mucous membrane is extremely tender
    d. Papulovesicular ulcers appear in the mouth and throat
    e. Submaxillary lymphadenitis is common
    f. Pain usually disappears 2 to 4 days before healing begins
    g. Lesions spread to the hand if thumb sucking is involved
  2. Aphthous stomatitis
    a. Burning, tingling, and slight swelling of the mucous membrane
    b. Single or multiple shallow ulcers with whitish centers and red borders appear and heal at one site, then reappear at another

C. Interventions
  1. Acute herpetic stomatitis
    a. Warm water mouth rinses; antiseptic mouthwashes are contraindicated because they irritate
    b. Topical anesthetic
    c. Bland liquid diet
    d. Rest
  2. Aphthous stomatitis
    a. Topical anesthetic
    b. Long-term; requires prevention of predisposing factors

◆ III. Esophageal diverticula

A. Pathophysiology
  1. Hollow outpouchings of one or more layers of the esophageal wall
  2. Occur in three main areas

Types of oral infections

DISEASE AND CAUSES	SIGNS AND SYMPTOMS	TREATMENT
Gingivitis (inflammation of the gingiva) • Early sign of hypovita- minosis, diabetes, blood dyscrasias • Occasionally related to use of oral contraceptives	• Inflammation with pain- less swelling, redness, change of normal contours, bleeding, and periodontal pocket (gum detachment from teeth)	• Removal of irritating factors (calculus, faulty dentures) • Good oral hygiene; regular dental checkups; vigorous chewing • Oral or topical cortico- steroids
Periodontitis (progression of gingivitis; inflammation of the oral mucosa) • Early sign of hypovita- minosis, diabetes, blood dyscrasias • Occasionally related to use of oral contraceptives • Dental factors: calculus, poor oral hygiene, malocclu- sion. Major cause of tooth loss after middle age	• Acute onset of bright red gum inflammation, painless swelling of interdental papillae, easy bleeding • Loosening of teeth, typi- cally without inflammatory symptoms, progressing to loss of teeth and alveolar bone • Acute systemic infection (fever, chills)	• Scaling, root planing, and curettage for infection control • Periodontal surgery to pre- vent recurrence • Good oral hygiene, regular dental checkups, vigorous chewing
Vincent's angina (trench mouth, necrotizing ulcerative gingivitis) • Fusiform bacillus or spiro- chete infection • Predisposing factors: stress, poor oral hygiene, in- sufficient rest, nutritional de- ficiency, smoking	• Sudden onset: painful, superficial bleeding gingi- val ulcers (rarely, on buccal mucosa) covered with a gray-white membrane • Ulcers become punched- out lesions after slight pressure or irritation. • Malaise, mild fever, ex- cessive salivation, bad breath, pain on swallowing or talking, enlarged sub- maxillary lymph nodes	• Removal of devitalized tis- sue • Antibiotics (penicillin or erythromycin by mouth) for infection • Analgesics, as needed • Hourly mouth rinses (with equal amounts of hydrogen peroxide and warm water) • Soft, nonirritating diet; rest; no smoking • With treatment, improve- ment common within 24 hours
Glossitis (inflammation of the tongue) • Streptococcal infection • Irritation or injury; jagged teeth; ill-fitting dentures; bit- ing during seizures; alcohol; spicy foods; smoking; sensi- tivity to toothpaste or mouth- wash • Vitamin B deficiency; ane- mia • Skin conditions: lichen planus, erythema multiforme, pemphigus vulgaris	• Reddened ulcerated or swollen tongue (may ob- struct airway) • Painful chewing and swal- lowing • Speech difficulty • Painful tongue without in- flammation	• Treatment for underlying cause • Topical anesthetic mouth- wash or systemic analgesics (aspirin and acetaminophen) for painful lesions • Good oral hygiene; regular dental checkups; vigorous chewing • Avoidance of hot, cold, or spicy foods, and alcohol

    a. Just above the upper esophageal sphincter (Zenker's diverticulum, the most common type)

    b. Near the midpoint of the esophagus (traction)

    c. Just above the lower esophageal sphincter (epiphrenic)

  3. Results from primary muscular abnormalities that may be congenital, or inflammatory processes adjacent to the esophagus

B. Assessment

  1. Midesophageal and epiphrenic diverticula with an associated motor disturbance (achalasia or spasm) seldom produce symptoms but may cause dysphagia and heartburn

  2. Zenker's diverticulum produces distinctively staged symptoms

    a. Throat irritation and regurgitation soon after eating

    b. Dysphagia and near-complete obstruction; regurgitation after eating may be delayed and may even occur during sleep, leading to food aspiration

  3. Hoarseness, asthma, and pneumonitis may be the only signs in elderly patients

  4. Chronic cough

  5. Bad taste in the mouth or foul breath

  6. Esophageal bleeding

C. Interventions

  1. Treatment for Zenker's diverticulum is usually palliative and includes a bland diet, thorough chewing, and drinking water after eating to flush out the pouched area or sac

  2. Severe symptoms or a large diverticulum necessitates surgery to remove the sac or facilitate drainage

  3. An esophagomyotomy may be necessary to prevent recurrence

  4. A midesophageal diverticulum seldom requires surgery except when esophagitis aggravates the risk of rupture; then treatment includes antacids and an antireflux regimen

    a. Keeping the head elevated

    b. Maintaining an upright position for 2 hours after eating

    c. Eating small meals

    d. Controlling chronic coughing

    e. Avoiding constrictive clothing

  5. Epiphrenic diverticulum requires treatment for accompanying motor disorders

    a. Achalasia, by repeated dilations of the esophagus

    b. Acute spasm, anticholinergic administration and diverticulum excision or suspending the diverticulum to promote drainage

  6. Depending on the patient's nutritional status, treatment may also include insertion of a nasogastric (NG) tube (passed carefully to prevent perforation) and tube feedings to prepare for the stress of surgery

◆ IV. Gastroesophageal reflux disease (GERD)

A. Pathophysiology

1. The backflow of gastric or duodenal contents, or both, into the esophagus and past the lower esophageal sphincter (LES), without associated belching or vomiting
2. Reflux may or may not cause symptoms or pathologic changes
3. Persistent reflux may cause reflux esophagitis (inflammation of the esophageal mucosa); the prognosis varies with the underlying cause
4. Causes
   a. Normally, the LES creates pressure, closing the lower end of the esophagus and preventing gastric contents from backing up into the esophagus then relaxing after each swallow to allow food into the stomach
   b. Reflux occurs when LES pressure is deficient or when pressure within the stomach exceeds LES pressure, allowing acidic stomach contents to pass back upward
   c. A person with symptomatic reflux cannot swallow often enough to create sufficient peristaltic amplitude to clear gastric acid from the lower esophagus; this results in prolonged periods of acidity in the esophagus when reflux occurs
5. Predisposing factors
   a. Pyloric surgery (alteration or removal of the pylorus), which allows reflux of bile or pancreatic juice
   b. Long-term NG intubation (more than 4 to 5 days)
   c. Any agent that lowers LES pressure, such as food, alcohol, cigarettes, anticholinergics (atropine, belladonna, propantheline), and other drugs (morphine, diazepam, calcium channel blockers, meperidine)
   d. Hiatal hernia with incompetent sphincter
   e. Any condition or position that increases intra-abdominal pressure, such as straining, bending, or coughing

B. Assessment

1. GERD doesn't always cause symptoms, and in patients showing clinical effects, physiologic reflux is not always confirmable
2. Most common feature of gastroesophageal reflux is heartburn, which may become more severe with vigorous exercise, bending, or lying down and may be relieved by taking antacids or sitting upright
3. Pain of esophageal spasm resulting from reflux esophagitis tends to be chronic and may mimic angina pectoris, radiating to the neck, jaws, and arms
4. Other signs and symptoms
   a. ODYNOPHAGIA, which may be followed by a dull substernal ache from severe, long-term reflux; dysphagia from esophageal spasm, stricture, or esophagitis

      b. Bleeding (bright red or dark brown)

      c. Rarely, nocturnal regurgitation wakens the patient with coughing, choking, and a mouthful of saliva

      d. Reflux may be associated with hiatal hernia; direct hiatal hernia becomes clinically significant only when reflux is confirmed

   5. Pulmonary symptoms result from reflux of gastric contents into the throat and subsequent aspiration

CLINICAL ALERT

      a. Chronic pulmonary disease or nocturnal wheezing, bronchitis, asthma, morning hoarseness, and cough

      b. In children, other signs consist of failure to thrive and forceful vomiting from esophageal irritation, which sometimes causes aspiration pneumonia

C. Interventions

   1. Effective management relieves symptoms by reducing reflux through gravity; strengthening the LES with drug therapy; neutralizing gastric contents; and reducing intra-abdominal pressure

   2. Drug therapy

      a. Antacids given at 1 and 3 hours after meals and at bedtime are effective for treating intermittent reflux; hourly administration is necessary for intensive therapy; a nondiarrheal, nonmagnesium antacid such as aluminum carbonate or aluminum hydroxide may be preferred, depending on the patient's bowel status

      b. Metoclopramide relieves gastric status by increasing LES sphincter tone and stimulating upper GI motility; omeprazole reduces gastric acidity

   3. Other measures

      a. If possible, NG intubation should not be continued for more than 5 days because the tube interferes with sphincter integrity and itself allows reflux, especially when the patient lies flat

      b. To reduce intra-abdominal pressure, the patient should sleep in a reverse Trendelenburg position (with the head of the bed elevated) and should avoid lying down after meals and late-night snacks

      c. In uncomplicated cases, positional therapy is especially useful in infants and children

   4. Surgery may be necessary to control severe and refractory signs and symptoms

      a. These include pulmonary aspiration, hemorrhage, obstruction, severe pain, perforation, incompetent LES, or associated hiatal hernia

      b. Surgical procedures create an artificial closure at the gastroesophageal junction

         (1) Belsey Mark IV operation (invaginates the esophagus into the stomach)

(2) Hill or Nissen procedures (creates a gastric wraparound with or without fixation)

(3) Vagotomy or pyloroplasty may be combined with an antire flux regimen to modify gastric contents

5. Teach the patient what causes reflux, how to avoid reflux with an antireflux regimen (medication, diet, and positional therapy), and what symptoms to watch for and report

6. For additional teaching tips, see *Patient with GERD*

◆ V. Gastritis

A. Pathophysiology

1. Inflammation of the gastric mucosa; usually self-limiting

2. Acute gastritis produces mucosal reddening, edema, hemorrhage, and erosion

   a. Chronic ingestion of irritating foods, caffeine

   b. Drugs: salicylates (containing aspirin); nonsteroidal anti-inflammatory drugs (NSAIDs)

   c. Ingestion of poisons

   d. Endotoxins released from infectious bacteria

3. Chronic gastritis is common among the elderly and persons with pernicious anemia (autoimmune gastritis)

   a. Commonly occurs as chronic atrophic gastritis, in which all stomach mucosal layers are inflamed, with reduced number of chief and parietal cells

   b. Results in atrophy of glandular epithelium; can become dysplastic and carcinomic

   c. May be associated with peptic ulcer disease or gastrostomy, chronic alcohol abuse, cigarette smoking, long-term use of NSAIDs

   d. Chronic reflux of pancreatic secretions, bile, and bile acids from the duodenum into the stomach

   e. Bacterial infection with *Helicobacter pylori* is a common cause of nonerosive chronic infectious gastritis

   f. Increased risk of peptic ulcer and gastric carcinoma

B. Assessment

1. Acute gastritis

   a. Rapid onset of symptoms

   b. Epigastric discomfort

   c. Indigestion

   d. Cramping

   e. Anorexia

   f. Nausea or vomiting

   g. HEMATEMESIS

TEACHING TIPS
Patient with GERD

Be sure to include the following topics in your teaching plan for the patient with gastroesophageal reflux disease (GERD):
• Instruct the patient to avoid circumstances that increase intra-abdominal pressure (such as bending, coughing, vigorous exercise, tight clothing, and constipation) as well as substances that reduce lower esophageal sphincter control (cigarettes, alcohol, fatty foods, caffeine, and certain drugs).
• Advise the patient to sit upright, particularly after meals, and to eat small, frequent meals.
• Tell him to avoid highly seasoned food, acidic juices, alcoholic drinks, bedtime snacks, and foods high in fat or carbohydrates, which reduce pressure on the lower esophageal sphincter.
• Advise the patient to eat meals at least 2 hours before lying down.
• Instruct the patient that obesity can increase intra-abdominal pressure. Assist with dietary planning.

    2. Chronic gastritis
       a. May have same symptoms as acute gastritis
       b. Mild epigastric discomfort
       c. May be asymptomatic or only have vague complaints such as intolerance to spicy or fatty foods or slight pain relieved by eating

C. Interventions
    1. Remove causative factors
    2. Treat chronic infectious gastritis with antibiotics
    3. Neutralize poisons with appropriate antidote
    4. Histamine-2 (H_2) receptor antagonists
    5. Antacids
    6. Vagotomy and pyloroplasty

◆ VI. Peptic ulcers

A. Pathophysiology
    1. Erosion of mucosal lining of the stomach and duodenum
    2. Imbalance between factors that promote inflammation and acid secretion (*H. pylori*, alcohol abuse, caffeine, smoking, prostaglandin inhibition) and factors that protect integrity of gastric and duodenal mucosa (mucosal secretions, alkali in duodenum)
    3. Possible etiology (see *How peptic ulcers develop,* page 160)
       a. Infection with *H. pylori*
       b. Alcohol abuse
       c. Stress (controversial)
       d. Drug induced: salicylates, steroids, indomethacin, reserpine

How peptic ulcers develop

Peptic ulcers can result from factors that increase gastric acid production or from factors that impair mucosal barrier protection. Infection with *Helicobacter pylori* underlies almost all peptic ulcer disease. Other factors increase mucosal injury.

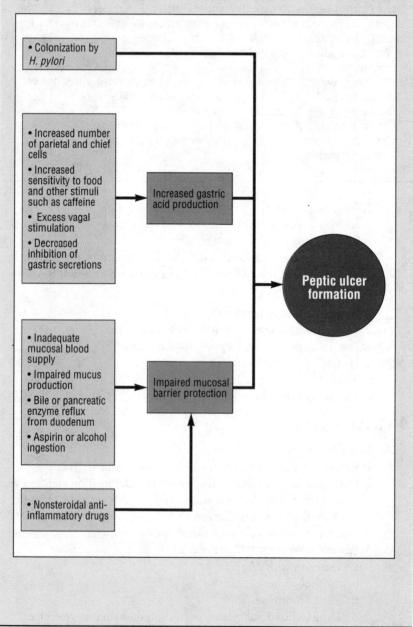

TEACHING TIPS
Patient with peptic ulcers

Be sure to include the following topics in your teaching plan for the patient with peptic ulcers:
• Teach the patient that chronic alcohol abuse, smoking, and use of some drugs (such as salicylates, nonsteroidal anti-inflammatory drugs, steroids) can cause peptic ulcer formation and exacerbation.
• Instruct the patient to take medications as prescribed. If indicated, this includes continuing to take antibiotics for the entire prescribed length of therapy.
• Encourage the patient to report any changes in his condition so that the doctor can tailor the treatment plan most effectively.
• Encourage the patient to eat four to six small meals daily.

   e. Increased gastric acid secretion (increased number of parietal cells)
   f. Smoking
   g. Gastritis
   h. Zollinger-Ellison syndrome

B. Assessment
   1. Epigastric pain on the left side 1 to 2 hours after eating; feeling of fullness after meals
   2. Weight loss
   3. Anorexia, nausea and vomiting
   4. Hematemesis
   5. MELENA
   6. Relief of pain after eating or taking antacids

C. Interventions
   1. Antibiotics to eradicate *H. pylori* (amoxicillin, tetracycline, clarithromycin, metronidazole)
   2. Diet: small, frequent feedings (4 to 6 meals/day); avoid whatever causes pain for the individual; also caffeine, smoking, alcohol (for additional teaching tips, see *Patient with peptic ulcers*)
   3. Proton pump inhibitors (omeprazole)
   4. Bismuth
   5. Prostaglandin analgesics (misoprostol)
   6. Sucralfate
   7. Antacids
   8. H_2-receptor antagonists
   9. Laser endoscopy
   10. Surgical intervention
      a. Subtotal gastrectomy
      b. Parietal cell vagotomy; truncal vagotomy and drainage, truncal vagotomy and antrectomy

◆ VII. Ulcerative colitis

A. Pathophysiology
1. Inflammatory disorder of the large bowel
2. Inflammatory edema of the mucous membrane of the colon and rectum leads to bleeding and shallow ulcerations
3. Abscess formation causes bowel-wall shortening, thinning, fragility, hypermotility, and decreased absorption
4. Mucosal ulcerations begin in the rectum and ascend the large intestine
5. Possible etiology
   a. Autoimmune disease
   b. Genetic factors
   c. Idiopathic
   d. Allergies
   e. Viral and bacterial infections
   f. Emotional stress
6. Increases risk of colon cancer by 10%

B. Assessment
1. Abdominal tenderness, distention
2. Bloody, purulent, mucoid, watery stools, 15 to 40/day
3. Weakness
4. Debilitation
5. Anorexia
6. Nausea and vomiting
7. Dehydration
8. Elevated temperature
9. Cachexia
10. TENESMUS
11. Hyperactive bowel sounds
12. Fever

C. Interventions
1. Diet
   a. High-protein, high-calorie, low-residue; bland foods in small, frequent feedings with restricted intake of milk and gas-forming foods
   b. Total parenteral nutrition (TPN) as needed
2. Semi-Fowler's position
3. Sitz baths
4. Medications
   a. Antibiotics such as sulfasalazine
   b. Corticosteroids
   c. Antiemetics
   d. Antidiarrheals
5. Surgery: colon resection, colectomy, or ileostomy (considered curative)

TEACHING TIPS
Patient with ulcerative colitis

Be sure to include the following topics in your teaching plan for the patient with ulcerative colitis:
• Emphasize to the patient that certain foods may make symptoms worse and that these foods should be avoided. Vomiting and diarrhea may cause loss of body fluids and electrolytes, and rapid movement of food through the intestines may cause deficiencies of fat, iron, calcium, and vitamins A, B_1, B_2, C, D, E, and K.
• Encourage the patient to report any changes in his condition so that the doctor can tailor the treatment plan most effectively.
• Tell the patient that he may be at risk for cancer, especially if the disease has persisted more than 10 years or since childhood.
• Explain the importance of adequate rest to the patient. To decrease intestinal motility during an attack, advise him to reduce physical activity. If his attack is mild, suggest that he rest more during the day.
• Advise him to avoid foods that irritate his intestines or that require excessive intestinal activity, such as milk products, spicy or fried high-residue foods, raw vegetables and fruits, and whole grain cereals. Explain that he may need supplemental vitamins to compensate for the bowel's inability to absorb them.
• Discourage carbonated, caffeinated, and alcoholic beverages because they increase intestinal activity. Also, discourage extremely hot or cold food and fluids because they cause gas.
• Advise eating small, frequent meals.

6. Electrolytes, and other fluid support as needed
7. Instruction in smoking cessation (for additional teaching tips, see *Patient with ulcerative colitis*)

◆ VIII. Crohn's disease

A. Pathophysiology
1. Inflammatory disease of unknown cause; affects small intestine; usually affects the terminal ileum; sometimes affects large intestine, usually the ascending colon
2. Slowly progressive disease with exacerbations and remissions
3. Ulceration of all layers of intestine, accompanied by congestion, thickening of the bowel, and fissure formations
4. Enlarged regional mesenteric lymph nodes accompany fibrosis and narrowing of intestinal wall
5. Possible etiology
   a. Genetic factors
   b. Allergies or immune disorders
   c. Infections
   d. Milk and milk products intolerance

        c. Fried foods

B. Assessment
1. Pain in right lower quadrant
2. Mesenteric lymphadenitis
3. Abdominal cramps and spasms after meals
4. Nausea
5. Flatulence
6. Weight loss
7. Elevated temperature
8. Chronic diarrhea
9. BORBORYGMUS
10. Blood in stools

C. Interventions
1. Diet: two types
   a. High-protein, high-calorie, low-residue, bland foods in small, frequent feedings with restricted intake of milk and gas-forming foods
   b. TPN as needed
2. Activity as tolerated
3. Medications
   a. Antibacterials
   b. Metronidazole
   c. Antacids
   d. Corticosteroids
   e. Immunosuppressants
   f. Antiemetics
   g. Antidiarrheals
   h. Anti–tumor necrosis factor
4. Surgery to correct bowel perforation, massive hemorrhage, fistulas, or acute intestinal obstruction
5. Refer patient to a support group such as the Crohn's and Colitis Foundation of America (for additional teaching tips, see *Patient with Crohn's disease*)

◆ IX. Irritable bowel syndrome (spastic colon)

A. Pathophysiology
1. A common condition marked by chronic or periodic diarrhea, alternating with constipation, and accompanied by straining (fecal urgency) and abdominal cramps or distention or both
2. A functional disorder that may be associated with stress
3. May result from physical factors
   a. Diverticular disease
   b. Ingestion of irritants such as coffee, raw fruits, or vegetables
   c. Lactose intolerance

TEACHING TIPS
Patient with Crohn's disease

Be sure to include the following topics in your teaching plan for the patient with Crohn's disease:
• Emphasize to the patient that certain foods may make symptoms worse and that these foods should be avoided. Vomiting and diarrhea may cause loss of body fluids and electrolytes, and rapid movement of food through the intestines may cause deficiencies of fat, iron, calcium, and vitamins A, B_1, B_2, C, D, E, and K.
• Encourage the patient to report any changes in his condition so that the doctor can tailor the treatment plan most effectively.
• Explain the importance of adequate rest to the patient. To decrease intestinal motility during an attack, advise him to reduce physical activity. If his attack is mild, suggest that he rest more during the day.
• Explain that dietary changes allow the bowel to heal by decreasing its activity while providing the calories and nutrition necessary for healing. Stress the importance of following his prescribed diet to help decrease symptoms.
• Advise him to avoid foods that irritate his intestines or that require excessive intestinal activity, such as milk products, spicy or fried high-residue foods, raw vegetables and fruits, and whole grain cereals. Explain that he may need supplemental vitamins to compensate for the bowel's inability to absorb them.
• Discourage carbonated, caffeinated, and alcoholic beverages because they increase intestinal activity. Also, discourage extremely hot or cold food and fluids because they cause gas.
• Advise eating small, frequent meals.
• If the doctor prescribes metronidazole to treat perianal complications of Crohn's disease, urge the patient to report any numbness or tingling in his extremities to his doctor immediately.
• Discourage smoking because it contributes to altered bowel motility.

---

   d. Abuse of laxatives
   e. Food poisoning
   f. Colon cancer

B. Assessment
   1. Low abdominal pain, usually relieved by defecation or passing of gas, and diarrhea that typically occurs during the day; these signs and symptoms alternate with constipation or normal bowel function
   2. Stools are commonly small and contain visible mucus; may be hard or watery
   3. Dyspepsia and abdominal distention may occur
   4. Fecal urgency

C. Interventions
   1. Avoid irritating foods; increase fiber (for additional teaching tips, see *Patient with irritable bowel syndrome*, page 166)
   2. Stress counseling
   3. Antispasmodics
   4. Rest

TEACHING TIPS
Patient with irritable bowel syndrome

Be sure to include the following topics in your teaching plan for the patient with irritable bowel syndrome:

• Caution the patient that he'll probably experience recurring bouts of irritable bowel syndrome if he doesn't follow prescribed treatment.

• Because the patient usually has a history of GI problems, instruct him to note and report any changes, including new or acute symptoms, unexplained weight loss, and hematochezia.

• Explain that long-term treatment consists of dietary management. Drug therapy is reserved for severe symptoms and is discontinued as patients make dietary and lifestyle changes and learn to manage stress.

• Explain that the GI tract works best on a schedule. And eating three meals daily of about the same volume, and at about the same time, and avoiding between-meal or late-night snacks promote regularity.

• Advise the patient to eat slowly and carefully to prevent swallowing air and consequent bloating.

• Suggest that the patient keep a daily record of food intake and symptoms. What foods appear to trigger symptoms? Advise him first to note them. Then he can proceed to eliminate them one at a time, thereby discovering which symptoms occur with certain foods.

• Explain that increasing dietary fiber can help relieve both diarrhea and constipation by adding essential soft bulk to stools. Inform the patient that constipation is controlled better by dietary fiber than by laxatives. Identify sources of dietary bulk, such as bran and other whole grain cereals, fresh fruit, and vegetables. Then propose ways to incorporate fiber into meals.

• Caution the patient to avoid fluids associated with GI discomfort, including carbonated and caffeinated beverages, fruit juice, and alcohol. But advise him to drink 8 to 10 glasses of compatible fluids daily to help regulate the consistency of his stools and promote balanced hydration.

• Advise your patient always to consult his doctor before treating constipation or diarrhea with over-the-counter medications because many irritate the bowel.

• Tell the patient to avoid alcohol and cold, allergy, and sleep medications, which may increase adverse reactions.

• Teach the patient that effective treatment may require lifestyle alterations that emphasize control of emotional tension. Be sure to help him set priorities by pinpointing the activities he enjoys, scheduling more time for rest and relaxation and, if possible, delegating responsibilities to other family members. If appropriate, encourage him to seek professional counseling for stress management.

• Teach the patient that regular physical exercise helps eliminate anxiety and promotes good bowel function.

• Discourage smoking because it contributes to altered bowel motility.

---

     5. Heat applied to abdomen

◆ X. Appendicitis

    A. Pathophysiology
       1. Inflammation of the appendix
       2. Most common major surgical emergency

3. Mucosal ulceration; exact cause of the ulceration is unknown, may be viral in nature
4. Inflammation accompanies ulceration and temporarily obstructs the appendix
5. Obstruction, if present, is usually caused by stool accumulation around vegetable fibers (fecolith)
6. Mucus outflow is blocked, which distends the organ
7. Pressure within the appendix increases
8. Bacteria multiply and inflammation and pressure continue to increase, affecting blood flow to the organ and causing severe abdominal pain

CLINICAL ALERT

9. Inflammation can lead to infection, clotting, tissue necrosis, and perforation of the appendix
10. If the appendix ruptures or perforates, the infected contents spill into the abdominal cavity, causing peritonitis
11. If untreated, appendicitis is fatal

B. Assessment
1. Abrupt onset of epigastric or periumbilical pain; as inflammation spreads, pain becomes more severe and localized in the right lower quadrant
2. Rebound abdominal tenderness and guarding
3. If the appendix is in the back of the cecum or in the pelvis, the patient may have flank tenderness instead of abdominal tenderness
4. Anorexia
5. Nausea or vomiting
6. Low-grade fever

C. Interventions
1. Appendectomy
2. Fluid and electrolyte replacement as indicated

◆ XI. Peritonitis

A. Pathophysiology
1. Localized or generalized inflammation of the serous membrane that lines the peritoneal cavity and covers visceral organs
2. Peritoneal irritants cause inflammatory edema, vascular congestion, and hypomotility of the bowel
3. Movement of extracellular fluid into the peritoneal cavity leads to hypovolemia and decreased urine output (third space fluid loss)
4. Possible etiology
   a. Bacterial infection
   b. Pancreatitis
   c. Blunt or penetrating trauma
   d. Inflammation of colon or kidneys
   e. Volvulus

      f. Necrosis or ischemia of intestine or gallbladder
      g. Intestinal obstruction or perforation
      h. Peptic ulceration
      i. Biliary tract disease
      j. Neoplasms
      k. Nephrosis
      l. Cirrhosis
      m. Pelvic inflammatory disease
      n. Abdominal surgery

B. Assessment
  1. Constant, diffuse, and intense abdominal pain
  2. Rebound tenderness
  3. Guarding
  4. Malaise
  5. Nausea or vomiting
  6. Elevated temperature
  7. Abdominal rigidity and distention
  8. Anorexia
  9. Decreased urine output
  10. Tachycardia, hypotension
  11. Shallow respirations
  12. Decreased peristalsis
  13. Decreased or absent bowel sounds
  14. Abdominal resonance and tympany on percussion
  15. Hiccup

C. Diagnostic tests
  1. Hematology: increased WBC count
  2. Peritoneal aspiration: positive for blood, pus, bile, bacteria, or amylase
  3. Abdominal X-ray: shows free air in abdomen, under diaphragm

D. Interventions
  1. Diet: TPN, no food or liquids
  2. NG tube for GI decompression
  3. Surgical intervention
  4. Antibiotics
  5. Analgesics
  6. Fluid and electrolyte replacement as indicated

POINTS TO REMEMBER

◆ Occult blood in stool and vomitus is a common finding in GI disorders.

◆ Pain from GI disorders may mimic angina pectoris.

♦ Appendicitis is the most common major surgical emergency.

STUDY QUESTIONS

To evaluate your understanding of this chapter, answer the following questions in the space provided; then compare your responses with the correct answers in appendix B, page 291.

1. Which foods should a patient with gastritis avoid? _____

_____

_____

2. Which part of the intestine is damaged in ulcerative colitis? _____

_____

_____

3. What are three possible causes of Crohn's disease? _____

_____

_____

4. What is the initial event in appendicitis? _____

_____

_____

CRITICAL THINKING AND APPLICATION EXERCISES

1. Observe a colonoscopy. Prepare an oral presentation for your fellow students, describing the procedure and the patient care required.

2. Interview a patient with ulcerative colitis. Evaluate the information for possible risk factors and identify ways to eliminate them.

3. Follow a patient with a GI disorder from admission to discharge. Develop a patient-specific plan of care, including any needs for follow-up and home care.

4. Develop a chart tracing the digestion of a meal.

Hepatobiliary Disorders

CHAPTER OVERVIEW

The liver is the largest and one of the busiest organs in the body, with over 100 separate functions. This remarkable, resilient organ serves as the body's warehouse and is absolutely essential to life. The gallbladder lies in the fossa on the underside of the liver and contains bile, which aids digestion.

Caring for the patient with a hepatobiliary disorder requires a sound understanding of the hepatobiliary anatomy and physiology. A thorough assessment is essential to planning and implementing appropriate patient care.

♦ **I. Liver**

    A. Structure

        1. Largest organ in the body

        2. Highly vascular; receives blood from two major sources, the hepatic artery and the portal vein

    3. Enclosed by Glisson's capsule, a network of connective tissue that covers the liver and extends into the parenchyma along blood vessels and bile ducts

    4. Located in the right upper quadrant of the abdomen, immediately below the diaphragm

    5. Divides into a right and left lobe, which are separated by a falciform ligament

    6. Small bile canaliculi fit between the cells in the cellular plates that radiate from a central vein and empty into terminal ducts; these ducts join two larger ones, which merge into a single hepatic duct upon leaving the liver.

    7. Hepatic duct then joins the cystic duct to form the COMMON BILE DUCT

B. Functions

    1. Carbohydrate metabolism; converts glucose to glycogen and stores it as fuel for the muscles

    2. Filters, metabolizes, and detoxifies blood, removing hormones, foreign substances such as drugs, alcohol, and other toxins

    3. Removes naturally occurring ammonia from body fluids, converting it to urea for excretion in urine

    4. Produces plasma proteins, nonessential amino acids, and vitamin A

    5. Metabolizes nutritional proteins

    6. Stores essential nutrients, such as iron and vitamins K, D, and B_{12}

    7. Produces bile to aid digestion

    8. Stores fat and converts excess sugars to fat for storage in other parts of the body

♦ II. Gallbladder

A. Structure

    1. Small, pear-shaped organ

    2. Located in the fossa under the liver

    3. Attached to the liver by connective tissue, the peritoneum, and blood vessels

    4. Divided into four parts:

        a. Fundus: broad inferior end

        b. Body: funnel shaped; bound to the duodenum

        c. Neck: empties into the cystic duct

        d. Infundibulum: lies between the body and neck; sags to form Hartmann's pouch

B. Functions

    1. Collects, concentrates, and stores bile

    2. Removes water and electrolytes from hepatic bile

    3. Increases the concentration of the larger solutes; lowers its pH below 7

4. Mild vagal stimulation causes the gallbladder to contract and Oddi's sphincter to relax and release bile into the duodenum

◆ III. Hepatitis

A. Pathophysiology

1. Viral inflammation of the liver due to direct cellular injury or secondary to the presence of an immune response that targets viral antigens on liver cells
2. Types of hepatitis
   a. Hepatitis A virus (HAV; formerly infectious hepatitis)
   b. Hepatitis B virus (HBV; formerly serum hepatitis)
   c. Hepatitis C virus (posttransfusion hepatitis)
   d. Hepatitis D virus
   e. Hepatitis E virus (see *Types of viral hepatitis,* pages 174 and 175)
3. Hepatitis B through E have been isolated in serum from patients with CRYPTOGENIC hepatitis
   a. Hepatitis F
      (1) Associated with enterally transmitted non-A-to-E hepatitis
      (2) Found in Central American population of Hispanic origin
   b. Hepatitis G
      (1) Structure resembles flaviviruses
      (2) Associated with parenteral transmission, especially patients undergoing hemodialysis and organ transplantation
      (3) Can infect the liver as an independent virus, but usually in the presence of hepatitis B or C
      (4) Minimal clinical impact with patients coinfected with hepatitis C virus; more severe liver damage when associated with HBV

B. Assessment

1. Preicteric phase
   a. Anorexia
   b. Nausea and vomiting
   c. Fatigue, malaise, or arthralgia
   d. Constipation or diarrhea
   e. Weight loss
   f. Right upper quadrant pain
   g. Hepatomegaly
   h. Splenomegaly
   i. Chills and fever
   j. Pharyngitis
   k. Nasal discharge
   l. Headache
   m. Pruritus

TEACHING TIPS
Patient with hepatitis

Be sure to include the following topics in your teaching plan for the patient with hepatitis:
• Advise the patient to avoid alcohol or other hepatotoxic agents.
• Advise the patient to avoid high-risk behaviors (I.V. drug use, unprotected sex).
• Encourage the patient to practice good personal hygiene.
• Instruct the patient to obtain follow-up testing for evidence of chronic state (if hepatitis B or C).
• Advise the patient that significant others, especially sexual partners (if hepatitis B) should be immunized.

2. Icteric phase
   a. Jaundice
   b. Worsening of prodromal symptoms with onset of jaundice
   c. Fatigue
   d. Weight loss
   e. Clay-colored stools
   f. Dark urine
   g. Hepatomegaly
   h. Splenomegaly
   i. Pruritus
3. Posticteric phase
   a. Fatigue
   b. Decreased hepatomegaly
   c. Decreased jaundice
   d. Improved appetite

C. Interventions
   1. Vaccination for HAV and HBV: immune globulin
   2. Diet: high-calorie, moderate-protein, high-carbohydrate, and low-fat
   3. Fluid and electrolyte replacement as needed
   4. Progressive, self-paced activity; avoidance of strenuous exercise
   5. For additional teaching tips, see *Patient with hepatitis*
   6. Standard precautions

◆ IV. Cirrhosis

A. Pathophysiology
   1. Chronic, progressive, irreversible disease
      a. Characterized by diffuse inflammation, fibrosis, and degeneration of hepatic cells

Types of viral hepatitis

The following chart compares the features of each type of viral hepatitis.

FEATURE	HEPATITIS A	HEPATITIS B
Incubation	15 to 45 days	30 to 180 days
Onset	Acute	Insidious
Age-group most affected	Children, young adults	Any age
Transmission	Fecal-oral, sexual (especially oral-anal contact), nonpercutaneous (sexual, maternal-neonatal), percutaneous (rare)	Blood-borne; parenteral route; sexual, maternal-neonatal; virus is shed in all body fluids
Severity	Mild	In many cases severe
Prognosis	Generally good	Worsens with age and debility
Progression to chronicity	None	Occasional

    b. Fibrotic tissue constricts flow in blood vessels and biliary ducts

2. Classified by cause
    a. Cryptogenic
    b. Alcoholic
    c. Virus induced
    d. Biliary
    e. Other rare forms
3. Inflammation destroys hepatic cells, with subsequent fibrosis
4. Fibrotic tissue changes obstruct hepatic blood vessels and bile ducts
5. Vascular obstruction causes portal hypertension; CHOLESTASIS causes hepatic cell necrosis
6. Decreased liver function impacts many other processes in body chemistry
    a. Impaired ability to convert ammonia to urea, to remove and conjugate bilirubin, and to synthesize bile
    b. Impaired gluconeogenesis
    c. Impaired metabolism of sex hormones
    d. Impaired synthesis of blood-clotting factors

HEPATITIS C	HEPATITIS D	HEPATITIS E
15 to 160 days	14 to 64 days	14 to 60 days
Insidious	Acute and chronic	Acute
More common in adults	Any age	Ages 20 to 40
Blood-borne; parenteral route	Parenteral route; most people infected with hepatitis D are also infected with hepatitis B	Primarily fecal-oral
Moderate	Can be severe and lead to fulminant hepatitis	Highly virulent with common progression to fulminant hepatitis and hepatic failure, especially in pregnant patients
Moderate	Fair, worsens in chronic cases; can lead to chronic hepatitis D and chronic liver disease	Good unless pregnant
10% to 50% of cases	Occasional	None

     e. Decreased absorption and utilization of fat-soluble vitamins (A, D, E, and K)

     f. Increased secretion of aldosterone

     g. Ineffective detoxification and metabolism of proteins, protein wastes, and poisonous toxins, especially alcohol

  B. Assessment

    1. Nausea and vomiting

    2. Weakness and fatigue

    3. Anorexia and weight loss

    4. Jaundice

    5. Ecchymosis

    6. Palmar erythema

    7. Indigestion

    8. Pruritus

    9. Irregular bowel habits, usually diarrhea

    10. Pain in right upper quadrant

    11. Peripheral edema, ascites, or both

    12. Petechiae

TEACHING TIPS
Patient with cirrhosis

Be sure to include the following topics in your teaching plan for the patient with cirrhosis:
• Keep nails short, avoid scratching.
• To relieve itching from jaundice, take cool-water baths, apply lotion containing lanolin.
• Eat a high-carbohydrate, low-fat, low-protein diet and minimize sodium intake.
• If portal hypertension is present, avoid activities that increase intra-abdominal pressure, such as heavy lifting, excessive coughing, straining at stool.
• Maintain safety in the home to avoid injuries that precipitate bleeding, and use assistive device when walking.
• If on diuretic therapy, monitor urine output, weigh daily, report signs of dehydration (thirst, decreased skin turgor, confusion).
• Maintain a semi-Fowler's position (head elevated 45 degrees) when resting.

---

13. Epistaxis
14. Hematemesis
15. Telangiectasis (caput medusae, "spider veins")
16. Gynecomastia and impotence
17. Amenorrhea
18. Hemorrhoids
19. Hepatomegaly, splenomegaly, or both
20. Melena
21. Esophageal varices
22. Encephalopathy with asterixis
23. Pleuritis, pericarditis

C. Interventions
1. Diet: high-calorie, high-carbohydrate, low-fat, low-sodium, low-protein in small, frequent feedings with restricted intake of alcohol and fluids
2. I.V. therapy; fluid and electrolyte replacement as needed
3. Semi-Fowler's position at rest
4. Diuretics, albumin
5. Stool softeners
6. Eliminate alcohol and other hepatotoxins
7. For additional teaching tips, see *Patient with cirrhosis*
8. Liver transplantation
9. Antibiotics such as neomycin
10. Treatment and monitoring of complications such as ascites, bleeding, and portal hypertension

◆ V. Liver abscess

A. Pathophysiology

1. Liver abscesses result when pyogenic or amebic organisms destroy hepatic tissue; resulting cavity fills with dead organisms, liquefied liver cells, and leukocytes; necrotic tissue walls off abscess from rest of liver

2. Relatively uncommon disorder

3. Mortality of 30% to 50%; increases to 80% if multiple abscesses

4. Pyogenic liver abscess

    a. The common infecting organisms are *Escherichia coli, Klebsiella, Enterobacter, Salmonella, Staphylococcus, Enterococcus,* and *Streptococcus*

    b. Organisms may invade the liver directly after a liver wound, or may spread from the lungs, skin, or other organs by the hepatic artery, portal vein, or biliary tract

    c. Generally multiple and commonly follow cholecystitis, peritonitis, pneumonia, and bacterial endocarditis

5. Amebic liver abscess

    a. Infection by *Entamoeba histolytica*

    b. Causes amebic dysentery

    c. Usually occurs singly in the right hepatic lobe

B. Assessment

1. Clinical manifestations depend on degree of involvement; some patients are acutely ill; in others abscess is found only at autopsy

2. Onset of symptoms usually sudden in pyogenic abscess; more insidious in amebic abscess

3. Signs and symptoms

    a. Right abdominal and shoulder pain

    b. Weight loss

    c. High fever

    d. Chills

    e. Diaphoresis

    f. Nausea and vomiting

    g. Anemia

    h. Jaundice

    i. Hepatomegaly

C. Interventions

1. Antibiotic therapy

2. Surgery usually avoided, but may involve drainage of abscess

3. Supportive care, based on symptoms

◆ VI. Cholecystitis and cholelithiasis

A. Pathophysiology
   1. Cholecystitis
      a. Inflammation of the gallbladder, acute or chronic
      b. Edema obstructs bile flow, which chemically irritates the gall-bladder
      c. Distention of organ may impair blood flow and deprive cells of oxygen-killing cells
      d. Dead cells slough off
      e. An exudate covers ulcerated areas, causing the gallbladder to adhere to surrounding structures
      f. Usually associated with a gallstone impacted in the cystic duct
      g. Surgery required in 10% to 25% of cases
   2. Cholelithiasis
      a. Stones (or calculi) in the gallbladder that result from changes in bile components
      b. Stones arise during periods of sluggishness in the gallbladder due to such conditions as pregnancy, diabetes, celiac disease, cirrhosis of liver, pancreatitis, and use of oral contraceptives
      c. Cholelithiasis accounts for 90% of all gallbladder and duct diseases

B. Assessment
   1. Acute abdominal pain in the right upper quadrant that may radiate to the back, between the shoulders, or to the front of the chest
   2. Pain commonly nocturnal or following meals rich in fats
   3. Recurring fat intolerance
   4. Biliary colic
   5. Belching
   6. Flatulence and indigestion
   7. Diaphoresis
   8. Nausea and vomiting
   9. Chills and fever
  10. Jaundice and clay-colored stools (if the stone obstructs the common bile duct)

C. Interventions
   1. Monitor vital signs and laboratory values
   2. Diet: low-fat
   3. Administer prescribed medications
      a. Vitamin K
      b. Antibiotics
      c. Analgesics
   4. Acute attack may require a nasogastric tube and I.V. line
   5. Nonsurgical removal of stones

    a. Insertion of catheter through a sinus tract into the common bile duct

    b. Endoscopic retrograde cholangiopancreatography

    c. Lithotripsy

    d. Stone dissolution therapy with oral chenodeoxycholic acid or ursodeoxycholic acid

6. Surgery: open or laparoscopic cholecystectomy

POINTS TO REMEMBER

♦ Hepatitis B is transmitted by blood and body fluids.

♦ Cirrhosis is characterized by irreversible chronic injury of the liver, extensive fibrosis, and nodular tissue growth.

♦ Cholecystitis may be induced by cholelithiasis (stone formation).

♦ A gallbladder ultrasound is used to visualize the gallbladder and locate obstruction by stones and is 96% accurate.

STUDY QUESTIONS

To evaluate your understanding of this chapter, answer the following questions in the space provided; then compare your responses with the correct answers in appendix B, page 292.

1. How are type A and type B hepatitis transmitted? _____

    _____

    _____

2. What are the common infecting organisms in pyogenic liver abscess? _____

    _____

    _____

3. What is the diet regimen for treating cirrhosis? _____

    _____

    _____

4. What surgical procedure is used in the treatment of cholelithiasis? _____

    _____

    _____

CRITICAL THINKING AND APPLICATION EXERCISES

1. Observe a gallbladder ultrasound procedure. Prepare an oral report for your fellow students, explaining the procedure and appropriate patient care.

2. Design a chart depicting how the gallbladder releases bile and its course.

3. Interview a patient with hepatitis. Evaluate the information for possible risk factors and identify ways to modify them.

4. Follow a patient with a hepatic disorder from admission through discharge. Develop a plan of care, including any needs for follow-up and home care.

Renal and Urologic Disorders

LEARNING OBJECTIVES
After studying this chapter you should be able to:
◆ Describe how the renal system functions.
◆ Differentiate between modifiable and nonmodifiable risk factors in the development of a renal or urologic disorder.
◆ List nursing interventions for a patient with a renal or urologic disorder.
◆ Identify three teaching topics to address for a patient with a renal or urologic disorder.

CHAPTER OVERVIEW

Together with the urinary system, the renal system serves as the body's water treatment plant. These systems work together to collect waste products from the blood and expel them as urine. They are also key to maintaining blood pressure, osmotic balances, hydrogen-ion concentrations, and other homeostatic mechanisms. Caring for a patient with a renal or urologic disorder requires a sound understanding of renal and urologic anatomy and physiology and mechanisms of fluid balance. A thorough assessment is essential to planning and implementing appropriate nursing care.

◆ I. Anatomy and physiology

A. Kidneys

1. Two bean-shaped organs located anterior and lateral to the 12th thoracic and first three lumbar vertebrae, behind the abdominal coelum and the peritoneum.
2. Four components: cortex, medulla, renal pelvis, NEPHRON
   a. Cortex
      (1) Makes up the outer layer of the kidney
      (2) Contains GLOMERULI; proximal tubules of the nephron; distal tubules of cortical and juxtaglomerular nephrons; and loops of Henle of cortical nephrons
   b. Medulla
      (1) Makes up the inner layer of the kidney
      (2) Contains loop of Henle of juxtaglomerular nephrons, and collecting tubules
   c. Renal pelvis: collects urine from the calices
   d. Nephron
      (1) Functional unit of the kidney
      (2) Contains the Bowman's capsule (glomerulus)
      (3) Contains the renal tubule, which consists of proximal convoluted tubule, loop of Henle, distal convoluted tubule, and collecting segments

B. Ureters

1. Ureters are a pair of fibrous, muscular tubes 11″ to 13.7″ (28 to 35 cm) long, which transport urine from the renal pelvis to the bladder
2. Ureterovesical sphincter prevents reflux of urine from the bladder into the ureter

C. Bladder

1. Muscular, distendable sac that stores urine
2. Total capacity of approximately 34 oz (1 L)

D. Urethra is a tube that transports urine from the bladder to the urinary meatus

E. Urine formation

1. Blood from the renal artery is filtrated across the glomerular capillary membrane in the Bowman's (glomerular) capsule
2. Filtration requires adequate intravascular volume and adequate cardiac output (CO)
3. Composition of formed filtrate is similar to blood plasma but without proteins
4. Formed filtrate moves through the tubules of the nephron and loop of Henle, which reabsorb and secrete electrolytes, water, glucose, amino acids, ammonia, and bicarbonate

5. Antidiuretic hormone and aldosterone control the reabsorption of sodium, potassium, and water

F. Blood pressure control
1. Regulation of fluid volume by the kidney affects blood pressure
2. Renin-angiotensin-aldosterone system (RAAS) is activated by decreased blood pressure and intravascular volume
3. Renal disease can alter the RAAS

G. Kidney synthesizes and secretes the hormone erythropoietin, which stimulates production of red blood cells (RBCs) in the bone marrow

H. Prostate gland
1. Surrounded by a fibrous capsule; connected to and surrounds the male urethra
2. Contains ducts that secrete the alkaline portion of seminal fluid and that open into the prostatic portion of the urethra

♦ II. Acute renal failure

A. Pathophysiology
1. Sudden interruption of renal function caused by obstruction, decreased perfusion, or nephrotoxins
2. Classifications include prerenal, intrarenal, and postrenal
3. Prerenal
   a. Results from conditions that diminish blood flow to the kidneys
   b. Azotemia (excess nitrogen, increased serum creatinine level) occurs in response to hypoperfusion; present in 40% to 80% of all cases of acute renal failure
4. Intrarenal
   a. Also called intrinsic or parenchymal renal failure; usually results in acute tubular necrosis (ATN)
   b. ATN accounts for approximately 75% of all cases of acute renal failure
   c. Prolonged ischemia or nephrotoxins injure the tubular segment
   d. Many possible causes of ischemic injury
      (1) Circulatory collapse
      (2) Severe hypotension
      (3) Dehydration
      (4) Trauma
      (5) Hemorrhage
      (6) Cardiogenic or septic shock
      (7) Surgery
      (8) Anesthetics
      (9) Transfusion reactions
   e. Nephrotoxic injury may be caused by ingesting or inhaling toxic chemicals; may also occur as a hypersensitivity reaction of the

kidneys to certain antibiotics or radiographic contrast agents; myoglobin or hemoglobin

  5. Postrenal
    a. Results from bilateral obstruction of urine outflow
    b. May be caused by prostatic hyperplasia or bladder outlet obstruction
  6. Each type of acute renal failure consists of three phases (oliguric, diuretic, and recovery)
    a. Oliguric phase
      (1) Decreased urine output (less than 400 ml/24 hours)
      (2) Kidney responds to decreased blood flow by conserving sodium and water, leading to volume overload
      (3) Electrolyte imbalances, such as hyperkalemia and metabolic acidosis
    b. Diuretic phase
      (1) Marked by increased urine output (more than 400 ml/24 hours
      (2) Caused by the kidney's inability to conserve sodium and water and by osmotic diuresis produced by high blood urea nitrogen (BUN) levels
      (3) Conditions may lead to deficits of potassium, sodium, and water; fatal if left untreated
      (4) Azotemia persists
    c. Recovery phase
      (1) Urine volume stabilizes
      (2) Azotemia resolves
      (3) Electrolytes normalize
      (4) 15% to 20% will progress to chronic renal failure and uremia

B. Assessment
  1. Related to changes in blood pressure and volume
    a. Oliguria
    b. Tachycardia
    c. Hypertension or hypotension
    d. Dry mucous membranes
    e. Flat neck veins
    f. Lethargy progressing to coma
    g. Decreased CO and cool, clammy skin in patients with heart failure
  2. Progression of renal failure may show signs and symptoms of uremia, including confusion, GI complaints, fluid in the lungs, infection, bleeding, pericarditis, and renal osteodystrophy

C. Interventions
  1. Encourage a high-calorie, low-protein, low-sodium, and low-potassium diet; restrict fluids

2. Monitor vital signs, intake and output, hemodynamic state, laboratory values
3. Monitor for signs of uremia
4. Administer prescribed medications
   a. Diuretics
   b. Electrolyte replacements, vitamin D
   c. Antibiotics
   d. Antihypertensives
   e. Erythropoietin
5. Dialysis
6. Fluid replacement as appropriate; hyperalimentation if catabolic weight loss is greater than 0.5 lb/day

◆ III. Acute pyelonephritis

A. Pathophysiology
1. Sudden inflammation caused by bacteria that affects the interstitial area and the renal pelvis or renal tubules
2. Infection usually spreads from the bladder to the ureters, then to the kidneys; may be spread hematogenously
3. Possible causes
   a. Congenital weakness at the junction of the ureter and bladder (vesicoureteral reflex)
   b. Instrumentation, catheterization, cystoscopy, or surgery
   c. Inability to empty the bladder; urinary stasis
   d. Urinary obstruction due to tumors, strictures, or benign prostatic hyperplasia

B. Assessment
1. Urgency, frequency, and burning during urination
2. Dysuria
3. Nocturia
4. Hematuria
5. Urine cloudy; may smell like ammonia or fish
6. Fever and shaking chills
7. Flank pain with radiation to labia or testes
8. Anorexia; nausea, and vomiting
9. General fatigue
10. Elderly patients: GI or pulmonary symptoms rather than the usual fever

C. Interventions
1. Observe urine appearance: send specimen for culture if appearance changes; also reculture 1 week after antibiotic therapy stops
2. Monitor vital signs, intake and output, and hemodynamic status
3. Administer prescribed medications
   a. Antibiotics

   b. Antipyretics
   c. Analgesics
  4. Surgery to relieve obstruction or correct anomaly
  5. Prevention of lower urinary tract infections

◆ IV. Acute poststreptococcal glomerulonephritis

A. Pathophysiology
  1. Also known as acute glomerulonephritis
  2. Relatively common bilateral inflammation of the glomeruli; usually follows a respiratory streptococcal infection or, less commonly, a skin infection such as impetigo, or infection with group A beta-hemolytic streptococcus
  3. Results from the entrapment and collection of antigen-antibody complexes in the glomerular capillary membranes, causing complement activation, which induces inflammatory damage and impedes glomerular filtration (type III hypersensitivity response)
  4. Damaged and inflamed glomerulus loses the ability to be selectively permeable and allow RBCs and proteins to filter through as the GFR falls
  5. Renal failure may result

B. Assessment
  1. History of streptococcal infection, usually pharyngitis or impetigo
  2. Mild to moderate edema
  3. Oliguria (urine output less than 400 ml/24 hours)
  4. Proteinuria
  5. Azotemia
  6. Hematuria (cola-colored urine), pyuria
  7. Fatigue
  8. Bilateral flank pain
  9. Mild to severe hypertension
  10. Heart failure due to pulmonary edema

C. Interventions
  1. Encourage a high-carbohydrate, high-vitamin diet with restriction of sodium, protein, potassium, and fluids
  2. Monitor vital signs, intake and output, and hemodynamic status
  3. Administer prescribed medications
   a. Antibiotics
   b. Antihypertensives
   c. Diuretics

◆ V. Renal infarction

A. Pathophysiology
  1. The formation of a coagulated, necrotic area in one or both kidneys that results from renal blood vessel occlusion

2. The occlusion reduces the rate of blood flow to renal tissues and leads to ischemia
3. Location and size of the infarct depends on the site of vascular occlusion; rate and degree of blood flow reduction determine whether or not the insult will be acute or chronic
4. Usually affects the renal cortex, but it can extend to the medulla
5. Usual causes
   a. Renal artery embolism secondary to mitral stenosis
   b. Infective endocarditis
   c. Atrial fibrillation
   d. Microthrombi in the left ventricle
   e. Rheumatic valvular disease
   f. Recent myocardial infarction

B. Assessment
1. Severe upper abdominal pain
2. Gnawing flank pain
3. Costovertebral tenderness
4. Fever
5. Anorexia
6. Nausea and vomiting
7. Renovascular hypertension
8. Acute renal failure (if both kidneys show significant infarction)

C. Interventions
1. Monitor vital signs, intake and output, and laboratory values
2. Encourage a low-sodium diet; monitor fluids
3. Administer prescribed medications
   a. Intra-arterial streptokinase
   b. Heparin therapy
   c. Antibiotics
   d. Antihypertensives
4. Catheter embolectomy
5. Surgical repair of occlusion or nephrectomy

◆ VI. Renal calculi

A. Pathophysiology
1. Also called kidney stones or nephrolithiasis
2. Form when substances that normally dissolve in urine precipitate
   a. Urine becomes concentrated with insoluble materials
   b. Crystals form and then consolidate forming calculi (see *How urine pH affects calculi formation,* page 188)
3. Calculi contain an organic mucoprotein framework and crystalloids
4. Mucoprotein is reabsorbed by the tubules, establishing a site for calculi formation

How urine pH affects calculi formation

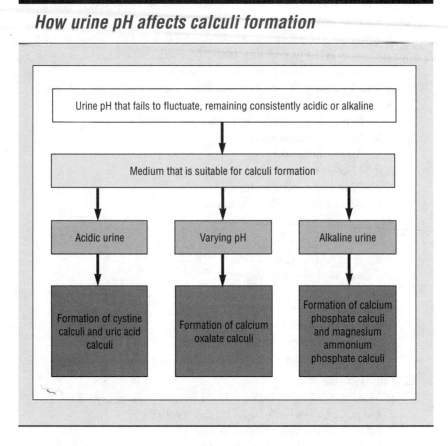

Urine pH that fails to fluctuate, remaining consistently acidic or alkaline

↓

Medium that is suitable for calculi formation

↓ ↓ ↓

| Acidic urine | Varying pH | Alkaline urine |

↓ ↓ ↓

| Formation of cystine calculi and uric acid calculi | Formation of calcium oxalate calculi | Formation of calcium phosphate calculi and magnesium ammonium phosphate calculi |

5. Calculi remain in the renal pelvis and damage or destroy kidney tissue or they enter the ureter
6. Large calculi in the kidneys may cause tissue damage
7. In certain locations calculi obstruct urine, which collects in the renal pelvis (these calculi tend to recur)
8. Initially, hydrostatic pressure increases in the collection system near the obstruction, forcing renal structures to dilate
9. With complete obstruction, pressure in the renal pelvis and tubules increases, the GFR falls, and a disruption occurs in the junctional complexes between tubular cells
10. If left untreated, tubular atrophy and destruction of the medulla leave connective tissue in place of the glomeruli, causing irreversible damage

CLINICAL ALERT

B. Assessment
1. Severe pain that spreads from the lower back to the sides and then to the pubic region and external genitalia; pain intensity fluctuates and may be excruciating at its peak

2. Constant dull pain
3. Nausea and vomiting
4. Fever and chills
5. Hematuria
6. Abdominal distention
7. Oliguria (bilateral obstruction in urine flow)

C. Interventions
1. Monitor vital signs, intake and output, and hemodynamic variables
2. Encourage large amount of fluid intake
3. Administer prescribed medications
   a. Antibiotics
   b. Analgesics
   c. Diuretics
4. Modify diet or urine pH based on specific diagnosis; encourage a low-calcium ion oxalate diet and daily ascorbic acid (to acidify urine), if indicated
5. Strain all urine
6. Cystoscopy, ureteroscopy
7. Lithotripsy
8. Nephrotomy

◆ VII. Nephrotic syndrome (NS)

A. Pathophysiology
1. Not a disease; a condition characterized by marked proteinuria, hypoalbuminuria, hyperlipidemia, and edema
2. Usually results from glomerulonephritis
3. Classifications
   a. Lipid nephrosis
      (1) Main cause of NS in children
      (2) Glomeruli appear normal
      (3) Some tubules may contain increased lipid deposits
   b. Membranous glomerulonephritis
      (1) Most common lesion in adult idiopathic NS
      (2) Characterized by uniform thickening of the glomerular basement membrane containing dense deposits
      (3) Eventually leads to renal failure
   c. Focal glomerulosclerosis
      (1) Can develop at any age, following renal transplantation, or result from heroin abuse
      (2) Lesions initially affect the deeper glomeruli, causing hyaline sclerosis, with later involvement of the superficial glomeruli
      (3) Slow, progressive deterioration in renal function

   d. Membranoproliferative glomerulonephritis
    (1) Slowly progressive lesions develop in the subendothelial re-
     gion of the basement membrane
    (2) May follow infection
  4. Other causes
   a. Metabolic disorders
   b. Circulatory diseases
   c. Nephrotoxins
   d. Allergic reactions
   e. Infections

B. Assessment
 1. Mild to severe dependent edema of the ankles or sacrum, or perior-
  bital edema; anasarca
 2. Orthostatic hypotension
 3. Lethargy
 4. Anorexia
 5. Depression
 6. Pallor
 7. Hematuria (rare)
 8. Oliguria may be present
 9. Ascites, pleural effusion

C. Interventions
 1. Correction of underlying disease
 2. Encourage a moderate-protein, low-sodium, low-fat diet
 3. Administer prescribed medications
  a. Diuretics
  b. Antibiotics
  c. Corticosteroids
 4. Monitor vital signs; watch for orthostatic hypotension
 5. Monitor for atherosclerotic phenomena; treat hyperlipidemia
 6. Weight-control diet
 7. Regular exercise program

◆ VIII. Chronic renal failure

A. Pathophysiology
 1. End result is tissue destruction and loss of kidney function
 2. Healthy nephrons compensate for destroyed nephrons by enlarging
  and increasing their CLEARANCE capacity; can maintain normal function until about 75% of nephrons are nonfunctional
 3. Eventually, the healthy glomeruli are so overburdened that they become sclerotic and stiff, leading to their destruction as well
 4. Progresses through four stages
  a. Reduced renal reserve: GFR is about 50% of the normal rate;
   asymptomatic

    b. Renal insufficiency: GFR is 20% to 50% of the normal rate; azotemia, anemia, hypertension

    c. Renal failure: GFR is 20% to 25% of the normal rate; azotemia, edema, metabolic acidosis, hyperkalemia

    d. End-stage renal failure: GFR is less than 20% of the normal rate; uremia present

  5. Possible causes

    a. Chronic renal disease that affects the capillaries in the glomeruli

    b. Chronic infection (chronic pyelonephritis or glomerulonephritis)

    c. Congenital anomalies

    d. Vascular diseases (such as hypertension)

    e. Obstruction

    f. Collagen diseases (such as systemic lupus erythematosus)

    g. Nephrotoxic agents

    h. Endocrine disorders (such as diabetes mellitus)

    i. Rapidly progressing disease of sudden onset that causes nephron destruction

B. Assessment

  1. Symptoms develop when more than 75% of glomerular filtration is lost; remaining normal tissue deteriorates rapidly

  2. Profound changes affect all body systems; major findings include:

    a. Hypervolemia

    b. Hyperkalemia

    c. Hypocalcemia, hyperphosphatemia

    d. Azotemia, oliguria

    e. Metabolic acidosis

    f. Anemia

    g. Peripheral neuropathy

  3. Other signs and symptoms by body system

    a. Cardiovascular: hypotension or hypertension, irregular pulse, life-threatening arrhythmias, hypervolemia, heart failure, edema

    b. GI: dry mouth, gum sores and bleeding, hiccups, metallic taste, anorexia, nausea, vomiting, ammonia smell to breath, abdominal pain on palpitation, diarrhea, GI ulceration

    c. Skin: loss of skin turgor; pallid, yellowish brown color; dryness; scaling; thin, brittle nails; brittle hair; severe itching; UREMIC FROST

    d. Neurologic: altered level of consciousness, listlessness, muscle cramps and twitching, pain, burning and itching in legs and feet

    e. Hematologic: GI bleeding and hemorrhage from body orifices, easy bruising, platelet abnormalities, anemia

    f. Musculoskeletal: fractures, bone and muscle pain, abnormal gait, impaired bone growth and bowed legs in children; fatigue

C. Interventions
1. Monitor vital signs, intake and output, laboratory values, and hemodynamic variables
2. Encourage a low-sodium, low-potassium, low protein, high-calorie, fluid-restricted diet
3. Administer prescribed medications
   a. Diuretics
   b. Digitalis glycosides
   c. Antihypertensives
   d. Antiemetics
   e. Iron, folate, and calcium supplements
   f. Synthetic erythropoietin
   g. Supplemental vitamins
   h. Antipruritics
   i. Phosphate binders
   j. Histamine blocker
4. Dialysis
5. Kidney transplant

Points to remember

◆ Renal disease can alter the renin-angiotensin-aldosterone system, which controls blood pressure.

◆ Specific gravity of urine, the patient's daily weight, and accurate fluid output measurements are important objective assessments for renal function.

◆ The nurse should observe the patient with acute renal failure for uremic frost.

◆ Major electrolyte imbalances can be life-threatening.

◆ Metabolic acid-base imbalances are caused by an underlying disease that disrupts the normal acid-base ratio.

Study questions

To evaluate your understanding of this chapter, answer the following questions in the space provided; then compare your responses with the correct answers in appendix B, page 292.

1. What are the three key functions of the renal system? _____

_____

_____

2. What is the most common cause of acute renal failure?_____

_____

_____

3. What does prerenal failure result from? _____

_____

_____

4. What is the cause of acute poststreptococcal glomerulonephritis? _____

_____

_____

5. What are two common causes of metabolic acidosis? _____

_____

_____

CRITICAL THINKING AND APPLICATION EXERCISES

1. Observe a dialysis treatment. Prepare an oral presentation for your fellow students, describing the procedure and patient care.

2. Develop a chart that depicts how fluid flows from the kidneys and is filtered to the bladder.

3. Interview a patient with a renal or urologic disorder. Develop a dietary plan that fits his or her illness and lifestyle.

4. Develop a chart comparing the major drugs used for treating hyperkalemia.

Endocrine and Metabolic Disorders

LEARNING OBJECTIVES

After studying this chapter you should be able to:

♦ Describe the role of the hypothalamus in regulating hormones.

♦ Explain how the pituitary gland, thyroid gland, adrenal glands, and pancreas function.

♦ Differentiate between modifiable and nonmodifiable risk factors in the development of an endocrine disorder.

♦ Identify the nursing interventions for a patient with an endocrine disorder.

CHAPTER OVERVIEW

Together with the central nervous system (CNS), the endocrine system regulates and integrates the body's metabolic activities and maintains homeostasis. Caring for the patient with an endocrine disorder requires a sound understanding of endocrine anatomy and physiology and fluid and electrolyte balance. A thorough assessment is essential to planning and implementing appropriate patient care.

◆ I. Anatomy and physiology

A. Hypothalamus

1. Produces hypothalamic-stimulating HORMONES, which affect the release and inhibition of pituitary hormones; also synthesizes vasopressin and oxytocin
2. Controls temperature, respiration, and blood pressure; food and water intake; and sexual activity
3. Affects the emotional states of fear, anxiety, anger, rage, pleasure, and pain

B. Pituitary gland

1. Considered the "master gland"
2. Consists of anterior and posterior lobes
   a. Posterior lobe stores and secretes vasopressin (antidiuretic hormone [ADH]) and oxytocin
   b. Anterior lobe synthesizes and secretes follicle-stimulating hormone, luteinizing hormone, prolactin, corticotropin, thyroid-stimulating hormone, and growth hormone
3. Factors altering pituitary gland function affect all hormonal activity

C. Thyroid gland

1. Accelerates cellular reactions, including basal metabolic rate and growth
2. Controlled by secretion of TSH from anterior pituitary
3. Produces thyroxine (T_4), triiodothyronine (T_3), and calcitonin

D. Parathyroid glands

1. Secrete parathyroid hormone (PTH), which regulates calcium and phosphorus metabolism
2. Require active form of vitamin D for PTH function

E. Adrenal glands

1. Adrenal cortex secretes three major hormone types
   a. Glucocorticoids (such as cortisol)
   b. Mineralocorticoids (such as aldosterone)
   c. Sex hormones (androgens, estrogens, and progesterone)
2. Adrenal medulla secretes two catecholamines
   a. Norepinephrine
   b. Epinephrine

F. Pancreas

1. Accessory gland of digestion
   a. Exocrine function: secretes digestive enzymes amylase, lipase, and trypsin
   b. Endocrine function: secretes hormones insulin, glucagon, and somatostatin from islets of Langerhans

2. Main pancreatic duct joins the common bile duct and empties into the duodenum at the ampulla of Vater

♦ II. Diabetes insipidus

A. Pathophysiology
1. Disorder of water metabolism caused by deficiency of ADH from the posterior pituitary or insensitivity of renal tissue to ADH
2. Absence of ADH allows water to be excreted in the urine instead of being reabsorbed in the renal tubules
3. Possible causes
   a. Drugs, such as lithium, demeclocycline
   b. Failure of the kidneys to respond to ADH
   c. Lesions of the hypothalamus, infundibular stem, and posterior pituitary

B. Assessment
1. Abrupt onset of extreme polyuria (usually 4 to 16 L/day of dilute urine, but sometimes as much as 30 L/day)
2. Polydipsia and consumption of extraordinarily large volumes of fluid
3. Weight loss
4. Dizziness
5. Weakness
6. Constipation
7. Increased serum sodium and serum osmolality levels

C. Interventions
1. Monitor vital signs, intake and output, and laboratory values
2. Replace fluids as ordered
3. Administer vasopressin as ordered
4. Treat the causative agent

♦ III. Hypothyroidism

A. Pathophysiology
1. Deficit of thyroid hormone T_3 or T_4, both of which regulate metabolism
2. Primary or secondary types
   a. Primary: stems from a disorder of the thyroid gland; may be iatrogenic (as in thyroidectomy ablation by radiation or drugs) or caused by other inflammatory conditions, chronic autoimmune thyroiditis, or iodine deficiency
   b. Secondary: stems from a failure to stimulate normal thyroid function due to lack of pituitary TSH

B. Assessment
1. Lethargy

TEACHING TIPS
Patient with hypothyroidism

Be sure to include the following topics in your teaching plan for the patient with hypothyroidism:
• Stress the need to take thyroid medication for life.
• Be sure the patient and family understand signs and symptoms of hypothyroidism and hyperthyroidism.
• Instruct the patient about the action, dosage, adverse effects, and specifics of administration of any thyroid medications; provide written instructions as appropriate.
• Encourage the patient to plan activities of daily living with adequate rest periods and to allow enough time for activities.
• Advise on the need for fiber and fluids in the diet to prevent constipation and on the need for daily exercise.

  2. Fatigue
  3. Forgetfulness, slow mentation, psychomotor retardation
  4. Sensitivity to cold
  5. Unexplained weight gain
  6. Constipation
  7. Anorexia
  8. Decreased libido
  9. Menorrhagia
 10. Paresthesia
 11. Joint stiffness
 12. Additional signs and symptoms related to specific body systems
    a. CNS: psychiatric disturbances, ataxia, intention tremor, carpal tunnel syndrome, benign intracranial hypertension, behavior changes
    b. Skin, hair, and nails: dry, flaky, inelastic skin; puffy face, hands, and feet; dry, sparse hair with patchy hair loss and loss of the outer third of the eyebrow; thick, brittle nails with transverse and longitudinal grooves; thick, dry tongue causing slow, slurred speech
    c. Cardiovascular: hypercholesterolemia with associated arteriosclerosis and ischemic heart disease, poor peripheral circulation, heart enlargement, heart failure, and pleural and pericardial effusions
    d. GI: achlorhydria, pernicious anemia, adynamic colon
    e. Reproductive: impaired fertility
    f. Eyes and ears: conductive or sensorineural deafness and nystagmus
    g. Circulatory: anemia

13. Myxedema: severe hypothyroidism
   a. Thickening of facial features
   b. Induration of the skin (myxedema)
   c. Rough, doughy skin
   d. Weak pulse; bradycardia
   e. Muscle weakness
   f. Sacral or peripheral edema
   g. Delayed reflex reaction time

C. Interventions
   1. Administer prescribed medications
      a. Thyroid hormone
      b. Iodine supplements
   2. Monitor vital signs and laboratory values
   3. Encourage high-fiber, high-protein, low-calorie diet with increased fluid intake
   4. For additional teaching tips, see *Patient with hypothyroidism,* page 197

◆ IV. Hyperthyroidism

A. Pathophysiology
   1. Metabolic imbalance that occurs when thyroid hormone is overproduced
   2. Excess thyroid hormone may cause various disorders
      a. Graves' disease
         (1) Most common hyperthyroid disorder
         (2) Autoimmune disorder that causes goiter, exophthalmos, dermopathy, and multiple systemic changes
         (3) Thyroid-stimulating antibodies bind and stimulate the TSH receptors of the thyroid gland
         (4) Caused by production of several autoantibodies formed because of a defect in suppressor T-lymphocyte function
      b. Other hyperthyroid disorders

**CLINICAL
ALERT**

         (1) Toxic adenoma: benign nodule that secretes thyroid hormone
         (2) Thyrotoxic crisis, also called thyroid storm: acute exacerbation of hyperthyroidism; rare, but it is a medical emergency
         (3) Thyrotoxicosis factitia: results from chronic ingestion of thyroid hormone for TSH suppression in patients with thyroid carcinoma
         (4) Functioning thyroid carcinoma
         (5) TSH-secreting pituitary tumor
         (6) Subacute thyroiditis: virus-induced inflammation of thyroid

B. Assessment
   1. Emotional stress
   2. Enlarged thyroid gland

TEACHING TIPS
Patient with hyperthyroidism

Be sure to include the following topics in your teaching plan for the patient with hyperthyroidism:
• Conduct an environmental assessment in the home to detect and correct potential injury hazards.
• Be sure the patient and family understand signs and symptoms of hypothyroidism and hyperthyroidism.
• Eat high-protein, high carbohydrate diet, in small frequent feedings, until ideal weight is achieved.
• Teach the patient to monitor radial pulse, and tell him what to report.
• Teach mode of action, adverse effects, dosage, and specifics of administration of any antithyroid medications.

3. Nervousness
4. Heat intolerance
5. Weight loss despite increased appetite
6. Excessive sweating
7. Diarrhea
8. Tremors
9. Thyroid hormones have widespread effects on all body systems
   a. CNS: difficulty concentrating, anxiety, excitability, fine tremor, shaky handwriting, emotional instability, mood swings, insomnia
   b. Cardiovascular: arrhythmias, cardiac insufficiency, cardiac decompensation, resistance to therapeutic dosage of a digitalis glycoside
   c. Skin, hair, and nails: vitiligo and skin hyperpigmentation; warm, moist skin with a velvety texture; fine, soft hair; premature graying; hair loss; fragile nails; onycholysis (separation of distal nail from nail bed)
   d. Respiratory: dyspnea on exertion
   e. GI: anorexia, nausea, vomiting, diarrhea
   f. Musculoskeletal: muscle weakness, generalized or local muscle atrophy, acropachy, osteoporosis
   g. Reproductive: menstrual abnormalities, impaired fertility, decreased libido, gynecomastia
   h. Eyes: infrequent blinking, lid lag, reddened conjunctiva and cornea, corneal ulcers, impaired upward gaze, convergence, strabismus, exophthalmos
C. Interventions
   1. Encourage high-protein, high-carbohydrate, high-caloric, diet with a restriction of stimulants

2. Monitor vital signs, intake and output, and laboratory values
3. Administer prescribed medications
   a. Antithyroid drugs
   b. Radioactive iodine
   c. Beta blockers
   d. Digitalis glycosides
   e. Glucocorticoids
4. Provide individualized home instructions (for teaching tips, see *Patient with hyperthyroidism,* page 199)
5. Surgical ablation
6. Fluids, glucose, and electrolytes replaced as needed

♦ V. Goiter

A. Pathophysiology
1. Enlargement of the thyroid gland not caused by inflammation or neoplasm
2. Two classifications:
   a. Endemic: caused by lack of iodine in the diet; leads to inadequate synthesis of thyroid hormone
   b. Sporadic: related to ingestion of certain drugs or food
3. Depletion of glandular organic iodine along with impaired hormone synthesis increases the thyroid's responsiveness to normal TSH levels
4. Resulting increases in both thyroid mass and cellular activity overcome mild impairment of hormone synthesis

B. Assessment
1. Single or multinodular, firm irregular enlargement of the thyroid gland
2. Stridor
3. Respiratory distress
4. Dysphagia
5. Dizziness or syncope when arms are raised above the head

C. Interventions
1. Encourage avoidance of goitrogenic foods, such as peanuts, peaches, peas, and strawberries; use iodized salt
2. Provide individualized home instructions
3. Administer thyroid replacement drugs and iodine as prescribed; avoid goitrogenic drugs such as cobalt, lithium, aminosalicylic acid, and propylthiouracil

♦ VI. Hypoparathyroidism

A. Pathophysiology
1. Deficiency of PTH

TEACHING TIPS
Patient with hypoparathyroidism

Be sure to include the following topics in your teaching plan for the patient with hypoparathyroidism:
• Teach the patient that chronic hypoparathyroidism is a lifelong problem.
• Be sure the patient and family understand signs and symptoms of hypocalcemia and hypercalcemia.
• Instruct the patient to return for follow-up serum calcium determinations.
• Advise the patient to follow a high-calcium, low-phosphorus diet.
• Teach mode of action, adverse effects, dosage, and specifics of administration of any calcium-, vitamin D–, or phosphate-binding medications.

2. PTH is not regulated by the pituitary gland or hypothalamus; it normally maintains blood calcium levels by increasing bone resorption, renal reabsorption, and GI absorption of calcium; also maintains an inverse relationship between serum calcium and phosphate levels by inhibiting phosphate reabsorption in the renal tubules
3. Causes
   a. Injury
   b. Idiopathy
   c. Magnesium deficiency
4. Classified as acute or chronic; acquired or idiopathic
   a. Acquired: commonly results from accidental removal or injury of one or more parathyroid glands during thyroidectomy or other neck surgery
   b. Idiopathic: may result from an autoimmune genetic disorder or congenital absence of the parathyroid glands

B. Assessment
1. Lethargy
2. Calcification of ocular lens
3. Muscle and abdominal spasms
4. Positive Trousseau's and Chvostek's signs
5. Numbness and tingling in fingers, lips, feet; carpopedal spasms
6. Arrhythmias
7. Seizures
8. Visual disturbances; diplopia, photophobia, blurring
9. Dyspnea
10. Laryngeal stridor or obstruction
11. Personality changes
12. Brittle nails
13. Alopecia
14. Deep tendon reflexes: increased

C. Interventions
1. Encourage high-calcium, low-phosphorus, low-sodium diet with spinach restriction
2. For additional teaching tips, see *Patient with hypoparathyroidism,* page 201
3. Monitor vital signs, intake and output, laboratory values, and ECG
4. Administer prescribed medications
   a. Calcium, vitamin D, magnesium
   b. Anticonvulsants
   c. PTH replacement
5. Provide respiratory support as needed

◆ VII. Hyperparathyroidism

A. Pathophysiology
1. Overactivity of one or more of the four parathyroid glands, resulting in oversecretion of PTH
2. Hypersecretion of PTH promotes bone resorption and leads to hypercalcemia and hypophosphatemia
3. Primary or secondary forms
   a. In primary disease, one or more of the parathyroid glands enlarges, increasing PTH secretion and elevating calcium levels; single adenoma is most common cause
   b. In secondary disease, excessive compensatory production of PTH stems from a hypocalcemia-producing abnormality outside the parathyroid gland; this causes a resistance to the metabolic action of PTH
   c. Hypocalcemia-producing abnormalities include rickets, vitamin D deficiency, chronic renal failure, or osteomalacia

B. Assessment
1. 75% of patients asymptomatic
2. Renal colic, renal calculi, hematuria, polyuria
3. Arrhythmias
4. Anorexia, nausea and vomiting, thirst, bowel obstruction, constipation, weight loss
5. Depression, mood swings
6. Slow mentation, paresthesia
7. Fatigue, muscle weakness
8. Osteoporosis, pathologic fractures, deep bone pain
9. Thickened nails

C. Interventions
1. Monitor vital signs, intake and output, laboratory values, and ECG pattern
2. Encourage a high-fiber, low-calcium, high-phosphorus diet in small, frequent feedings, with an increase in fluid intake (I.V. hydration as needed)

3. Administer prescribed medications
   a. Diuretics (not loop or thiazide diuretics)
   b. Analgesics
   c. Estrogen
   d. Biphosphonates
   e. Antineoplastics
   f. Calcitonin
   g. Propranolol
4. Radiation therapy
5. Dialysis
6. Parathyroidectomy

◆ VIII. Adrenal insufficiency

A. Pathophysiology
1. Also called Addison's disease, adrenal hypofunction, or adrenal insufficiency
2. Primary or secondary forms
   a. Primary
      (1) Originates within the adrenal glands
      (2) Characterized by decreased mineralocorticoid, glucocorticoid, and androgen secretion
      (3) More than 90% of both adrenal glands are destroyed
      (4) Addison's disease is most common form
   b. Secondary
      (1) Caused by a disorder outside the adrenal gland
      (2) Aldosterone secretion may be unaffected
3. Causes
   a. Primary
      (1) Tuberculosis
      (2) Removal of both adrenal glands
      (3) Hemorrhage into the adrenal gland
      (4) Neoplasms
      (5) Infections; autoimmune process
      (6) Acquired immunodeficiency syndrome
   b. Secondary
      (1) Hypopituitarism (trauma, surgery, tumor, and radiation): may lead to decreased corticotropin secretion
      (2) Removal of a nonendocrine corticotropin-secreting tumor
      (3) Disorders in hypothalamic-pituitary function that diminish the production of corticotropin

CLINICAL ALERT

4. Adrenal crisis
   a. Also called Addisonian crisis
   b. Critical deficiency of mineralocorticoids and glucocorticoids
   c. Rare, but a medical emergency that requires immediate, vigorous treatment

B. Assessment
1. Hypoglycemia
2. Weakness and lethargy; confusion
3. Bronzed skin pigmentation of nipples, scars, and buccal mucosa (with corticotropin excess)
4. Dehydration
5. Anorexia
6. Thirst
7. Decreased pubic and axillary hair in women
8. Hypotension
9. Diarrhea
10. Nausea
11. Weight loss
12. Depression or emotional lability
13. Abdominal pain
14. Headache
15. Fever

C. Interventions
1. Monitor vital signs, intake and output, laboratory values, and ECG pattern
2. Encourage a high-carbohydrate, high-protein, high-sodium, low-potassium diet prior to steroid therapy; high-potassium, low-sodium diet when on steroid therapy
3. Administer prescribed medications
   a. Vasopressors
   b. Antacids
   c. Mineralocorticoids
   d. Glucocorticoids
4. Replace fluids (I.V. saline) electrolytes, and glucose, as needed
5. Chemotherapy, radiation, or surgery for pituitary tumor

◆ IX. Cushing's syndrome

A. Pathophysiology
1. Presence of excessive glucocorticoids (hypercortisolism) for any reason
2. Primary, secondary, tertiary, and iatrogenic forms
   a. Primary: caused by a disease of the adrenal cortex; usually an adrenal tumor
   b. Secondary: caused by hyperfunction of corticotropin-secreting cells of the anterior pituitary (Cushing's *disease*); usually pituitary adenoma; may also involve increased corticotropin from ectopic source, such as a lung tumor
   c. Tertiary: caused by hypothalamic dysfunction or injury

TEACHING TIPS
Patient with Cushing's syndrome

Be sure to include the following topics in your teaching plan for the patient with Cushing's syndrome:
• Tell the patient to avoid crowds or individuals with respiratory or other infections; stress proper handwashing techniques.
• Be sure the patient and family understand signs and symptoms of hypocalcemia and hypercalcemia.
• Encourage the patient to maintain weight reduction program to achieve an ideal weight; advise him or her to walk and regularly exercise.
• Instruct the patient to follow a low-sodium, high-protein diet.
• Reinforce the need for lifelong follow-up and the importance of wearing a medical identification bracelet.

    d. Iatrogenic: caused by long-term therapy with EXOGENOUS corticosteroids

B. Assessment
1. Cervicodorsal fat pads (buffalo hump)
2. Thinning extremities with muscle wasting and fat mobilization to trunk (truncal obesity)
3. Moon face and ruddy complexion
4. Hirsutism
5. Broad purple striae
6. Bruising
7. Impaired wound healing
8. Osteoporosis
9. Thinning hair (baldness)
10. Hypertension
11. Fatigue
12. Amenorrhea or oligomenorrhea
13. Impotence
14. Hyperglycemia

C. Interventions
1. Monitor vital signs, intake and output, laboratory values
2. Encourage a low-sodium, low-carbohydrate, low-calorie, high-potassium, and high-protein diet
3. For additional teaching tips, see *Patient with Cushing's syndrome*
4. Administer prescribed medications
    a. Diuretics
    b. Potassium supplements
    c. Adrenal suppressants (such as ketoconazole, metyrapone, aminoglutethimide)

d. Antidiabetic drugs
5. Radiation: pituitary gland
6. Surgery: pituitary gland or adrenal cortex

◆ X. Diabetes mellitus

A. Pathophysiology
1. Chronic disease of insulin deficiency or resistance that blocks tissues' access to essential nutrients for fuel and storage
   a. Insulin allows glucose to travel into cells to be used for energy and stored as glycogen
   b. Insulin stimulates protein synthesis and free fatty acid storage in adipose tissue
2. Four types, classified by etiology
   a. Type 1: further subdivided into immune-mediated diabetes and idiopathic diabetes
      (1) Beta cells in the pancreas are destroyed or suppressed, resulting in a failure to release insulin and ineffective glucose transport
      (2) Immune-mediated diabetes is caused by cell-mediated destruction of pancreatic beta cells; rate of beta cell destruction is usually higher in children than in adults
      (3) By the time the disease becomes apparent, 80% of beta cells are gone
      (4) Idiopathic type 1 diabetes has no known cause; patients with this form have no evidence of autoimmunity and do not produce insulin
   b. Type 2: (more prevalent form), beta cells release insulin, but receptors are insulin-resistant and glucose transport is variable and ineffective; numerous risk factors
      (1) Obesity (risk decreases with weight loss and drug therapy)
      (2) Lack of physical activity
      (3) History of gestational diabetes
      (4) Hypertension or dyslipidemia
      (5) Black, Hispanic, or Native American origin
      (6) Strong family history of diabetes
      (7) Advancing age
   c. Gestational diabetes mellitus
      (1) Occurs during pregnancy
      (2) May result from weight gain and increased levels of estrogen and placental hormones, which antagonize insulin
      (3) Glucose tolerance levels usually return to normal after delivery
   d. Other specific types

Understanding DKA and HHNS

Diabetic ketoacidosis (DKA) and hyperosmolar hyperglycemic nonketotic syndrome (HHNS) are acute complications of hyperglycemic crises that may occur with diabetes. If not treated properly, either may result in coma or death.

DKA usually occurs with type 1 diabetes and may be the first evidence of the disease. HHNS usually occurs in patients with type 2 diabetes, but it also occurs in anyone whose insulin tolerance is stressed and in patients who've undergone certain therapeutic procedures, such as peritoneal dialysis, hemodialysis, tube feedings, or total parenteral nutrition.

Acute insulin deficiency (absolute DKA; relative in HHNS) precipitates both conditions. Causes include illness, stress, infection and in patients with DKA, failure to take insulin.

Buildup of glucose

Inadequate insulin hinders glucose uptake by fat and muscle cells. Because the cells can't take in glucose to convert to energy, glucose accumulates in the blood. At the same time, the liver responds to the demands of the energy-starved cells by converting glycogen to glucose and releasing glucose into the blood, further increasing the blood glucose level. When this level exceeds the renal threshold, excess glucose is excreted in the urine.

Still, the insulin-deprived cells can't use glucose. Their response is rapid metabolism of protein, which results in loss of intracellular potassium and phosphorus and excessive liberation of amino acids. The liver converts these amino acids into urea and glucose.

As a result of these processes, blood glucose levels are grossly elevated. The aftermath is increased serum osmolarity and glycosuria (high amounts of glucose in the urine), leading to osmotic diuresis. Glycosuria is higher in HHNS than in DKA because blood glucose levels are higher in HHNS.

A deadly cycle

The massive fluid loss from osmotic diuresis causes fluid and electrolyte imbalances and dehydration. Water loss exceeds glucose and electrolyte loss, contributing to hyperosmolarity. This, in turn, perpetuates dehydration, decreasing the glomerular filtration rate and reducing the amount of glucose excreted in the urine. This leads to a deadly cycle: diminished glucose excretion further raises blood glucose levels, producing hyperosmolarity and finally causing shock, coma, and death.

DKA complication

All of these steps hold true for both DKA and HHNS, but DKA involves an additional, simultaneous process that leads to metabolic acidosis. The absolute insulin deficiency causes cells to convert fats into glycerol and fatty acids for energy. The fatty acids can't be metabolized as quickly as they're released, so they accumulate in the liver, where they're converted into ketones (keto acids). These ketones accumulate in the blood and urine and cause acidosis. Acidosis leads to more tissue breakdown, more ketosis, more acidosis, and eventually shock, coma, and death.

TEACHING TIPS
Patient with diabetes mellitus

Be sure to include the following topics in your teaching plan for the patient with diabetes mellitus:
• Arrange for individualized home instruction.
• Provide information about the American Diabetes Association.
• Discuss the need for maintaining normal weight.
• Review the procedure for fingerstick blood glucose monitoring.
• Emphasize the importance of frequent blood glucose monitoring.
• Review insulin requirements and administration technique.
• Discuss insulin's action, dosage, frequency, and possible effects.
• Emphaszie possible danger signs (hyperglycemia or hypoglycemia).
• Review dietary restrictions.
• Caution a pregnant patient about implications for the mother and fetus.
• Remind the patient of activity and exercise precautions and sick-day regimen.
• Advise the patient about regular checkups and diagnostic testing.
• Explain the need for meticulous foot care.
• Emphasize the need for compliance and follow-up care.

CLINICAL ALERT

    (1) Includes people who have diabetes as a result of a genetic defect of the beta cells or endocrinopathies
    (2) Exposure to certain drugs or chemicals
  3. Acute complications: diabetic ketoacidosis (DKA) and hyperosmolar hyperglycemic nonketotic syndrome (HHNS); both require immediate medical intervention (see *Understanding DKA and HHNS,* page 207)

B. Assessment
  1. Weight loss
  2. Polyphagia (early sign)
  3. Abdominal cramping, nausea, vomiting, anorexia
  4. Acetone breath
  5. Weakness
  6. Fatigue
  7. Dehydration
  8. Pain
  9. Paresthesia
  10. Polyuria
  11. Polydipsia
  12. Kussmaul's respirations
  13. Multiple infections and boils
  14. Flushed, warm, smooth, shiny skin
  15. Atrophic muscles
  16. Poor wound healing

17. Mottled extremities
18. Peripheral and visceral neuropathies
19. Retinopathy or nephropathy, or both
20. Blurred vision
21. Sexual dysfunction
22. Macrovascular and microvascular disease (long-term)

C. Interventions
1. Monitor vital signs, intake and output, laboratory values
2. Encourage prescribed diet based on metabolic activity, ideal weight, and personal activity
3. For additional teaching tips, see *Patient with diabetes mellitus*
4. Administer prescribed medications
   a. Antidiabetic drugs or insulin (intermittent or continuous I.V. or subcutaneous infusion), based on frequent blood glucose assessments
   b. Vitamin and mineral supplements
5. Pancreas transplant

◆ XI. Porphyria

A. Pathophysiology
1. Group of inherited metabolic disorders that affect the biosynthesis of heme and cause excessive production and excretion of porphyrins or their precursors
2. Porphyrins, present in all protoplasm, figure prominently in energy storage and use
3. Classification depends on the site of excessive porphyrin production (see *Types of porphyria*, page 210)
   a. Erythropoietic: erythmoid cells in bone marrow
   b. Hepatic: liver
   c. Erythrohepatic: in bone marrow and liver
4. Possible causes
   a. Inherited as autosomal dominant traits
   b. Autosomal recessive trait: Gunther's disease
   c. Toxic: acquired (usually from lead ingestion)

B. Assessment
1. Photosensitivity
2. Facial hirsutism, blistering, edema
3. Acute abdominal pain
4. Neuropathy
5. Complex syndrome (hepatic porphyrias)
   a. Chronic brain syndrome, seizures
   b. Peripheral neuropathy
   c. Tachycardia
   d. Labile hypertension

Types of porphyria

PORPHYRIA	SIGNS AND SYMPTOMS	TREATMENT
Erythropoietic porphyria		
Günther's disease • Usual onset before age 5	• Red urine (earliest, most characteristic sign); severe cutaneous photosensitivity, leading to vesicular or bullous eruptions on exposed areas and, eventually, scarring and ulceration • Hypertrichosis • Brown-stained or red-stained teeth • Splenomegaly, hemolytic anemia	• Beta-carotene by mouth to prevent photosensitivity reactions • Anti-inflammatory ointments • Prednisone to reverse anemia • Packed red cells to inhibit erythropoiesis and excreted porphyrins • Hemin for recurrent attacks • Splenectomy for hemolytic anemia • Topical dihydroxyacetone and lawsone sunscreen filter
Erythrohepatic porphyria		
Protoporphyria • Usually affects children • Usually occurs in males	• Photosensitive dermatitis • Hemolytic anemia • Chronic hepatic disease	• Avoidance of causative factors • Beta-carotene to reduce photosensitivity
Toxic-acquired porphyria • Usually affects children • Significant mortality	• Acute colicky pain • Anorexia, nausea, vomiting • Neuromuscular weakness • Behavioral changes • Seizures, coma	• Chlorpromazine I.V. to relieve pain and GI symptoms • Avoidance of lead exposure
Acute intermittent porphyria • Most common form • Usually affects females between ages 15 and 40	• Colicky abdominal pain with fever, general malaise, and hypertension • Peripheral neuritis, behavioral changes, possibly leading to frank psychosis • Respiratory paralysis can occur	• Chlorpromazine I.V. to relieve abdominal pain and control psychic abnormalities • Avoidance of barbiturates, infections, alcohol, and fasting • Hemin for recurrent attacks • High-carbohydrate diet
Hepatic porphyria		
Variegate porphyria • Usual onset between ages 30 and 50 • Occurs almost exclusively among South African whites • Affects males and females equally	• Skin lesions, extremely fragile skin in exposed areas • Hypertrichosis • Hyperpigmentation • Abdominal pain during acute attack • Neuropsychiatric manifestations	• High-carbohydrate diet • Avoidance of sunlight, or wearing of protective clothing when avoidance isn't possible • Hemin for recurrent attacks
Porphyria cutanea tarda • Most common in men ages 40 to 60 • Highest incidence in South Africans	• Facial pigmentation • Red-brown urine • Photosensitive dermatitis • Hypertrichosis	• Avoidance of precipitating factors, such as alcohol and estrogens • Phlebotomy at 2-week intervals to lower serum iron level
Hereditary coproporphyria • Rare • Affects males and females equally	• Asymptomatic or mild neurologic, abdominal, or psychiatric symptoms	• High-carbohydrate diet • Avoidance of barbiturates • Hemin for recurrent attacks

TEACHING TIPS
Patient with porphyria

Be sure to include the following topics in your teaching plan for the patient with porphyria:
• Avoid crowds or individuals with respiratory or other infections; stress proper hand washing.
• Avoid factors, especially drugs, capable of precipitating attacks.
• Refer the patient for genetic counseling as needed.
• Follow high-carbohydrate diet.
• Reinforce the need for lifelong follow-up.
• Wear medical identification bracelet.

     e. Severe colicky lower abdominal pain, vomiting
     f. Constipation
     g. Itching and burning from skin lesions
     h. Altered pigmentation and edema in areas exposed to light

C. Interventions
    1. Genetic counseling
    2. Teach to avoid overexposure to the sun and use of beta-carotene to reduce photosensitivity; avoid factors that precipitate attacks
    3. Acute attacks: analgesics, I.V. glucose, and hematin
    4. Encourage a high-carbohydrate diet with restricted fluid intake
    5. For additional teaching tips, see *Patient with porphyria*

POINTS TO REMEMBER

◆ Factors altering the function of the pituitary gland—the master gland—affect all of the body's hormonal activity.

◆ All four parathyroid glands secrete PTH, the principle regulator of calcium metabolism.

◆ Diabetes insipidus causes excessive urination and excessive thirst and fluid intake.

◆ Two acute metabolic complications of diabetes mellitus are DKA and HHNS; both are life-threatening.

STUDY QUESTIONS

To evaluate your understanding of this chapter, answer the following questions in the space provided; then compare your responses with the correct answers in appendix B, pages 292 and 293.

1. What are possible assessment findings for hypothyroidism?_____

_____

_____

2. What is Graves' disease? _____

_____

_____

3. What are three symptoms of Addison's disease?_____

_____

_____

4. What causes Cushing's syndrome?_____

_____

_____

5. What are the four types of diabetes mellitus?_____

_____

_____

CRITICAL THINKING AND APPLICATION EXERCISES

1. Observe a glucose tolerance test. Prepare an oral presentation for your fellow students describing the procedure and patient care.

2. Obtain a dietary history from a patient with diabetes. Using the patient's prescribed meal plan, assist him in choosing meals from the exchange list provided by the American Diabetes Association.

3. Follow a patient with an endocrine disorder from admission through discharge. Develop a patient-specific plan of care, including any needs for follow-up and home care.

Male reproductive disorders

LEARNING OBJECTIVES

After studying this chapter, you should be able to:

♦ Describe how pathogens are spread in prostatitis.

♦ Discuss assessment findings in acute, chronic, and nonbacterial prostatitis.

♦ Determine nursing interventions for the patient with epididymitis.

♦ Discuss a clinical finding to watch for with epididymitis.

♦ Discuss the probable causes of benign prostatic hyperplasia.

♦ Assess and plan care for a male patient with a reproductive system disorder.

CHAPTER OVERVIEW

The male reproductive system (penis, epididymis, prostate, and two testicles suspended in the scrotum) is so closely involved with the urinary system that disease in one system often causes symptoms in the other. Knowledge of male reproductive and urinary system function helps the nurse understand conditions associated with altered reproductive system function. Thorough assessment is essential for diagnosis and early treatment to prevent long-term and chronic conditions from occurring.

♦ I. Types of disorders

A. Infectious disorders
  1. Three causes of infectious disorders
     a. Sexually transmitted diseases
     b. Systemic infections
     c. Instrumentation (iatrogenic)
  2. Affect any or all parts of the male reproductive system
  3. May impact both sexual function and reproductive ability

B. Prostate disorders result from enlargement or infection of the prostate gland

C. Neoplasms include prostate cancer (see chapter 19), testicular cancer, and penile cancer

D. Congenital disorders usually result from a structural malformation of the penis or testes (hypospadias, epispadias) and may affect urinary or reproductive function

♦ II. Prostatitis

A. Pathophysiology
  1. An acute or chronic bacterial or nonbacterial inflammation of the prostate gland
  2. About 80% of bacterial prostatitis cases result from *Escherichia coli* infection
  3. Remaining 20% are caused by *Klebsiella, Enterobacter, Proteus, Pseudomonas, Serratia, Streptococcus, Staphylococcus,* and diphtheroids
  4. Causative organisms probably spread to the prostate by one of four pathways
     a. The bloodstream
     b. Ascending urethral infection
     c. Invasion by rectal bacteria through lymphatic vessels
     d. Reflux of infected urine from the bladder into prostatic ducts
  5. Chronic bacterial prostatitis is usually caused by bacterial invasion from the urethra
  6. Less common means of infection are secondary to cystoscopy, or urethral catheterization; also from infrequent (or excessive) sexual intercourse
  7. Nonbacterial prostatitis cause is unknown

B. Assessment
  1. Acute prostatitis
     a. Fever
     b. Chills
     c. MYALGIA, malaise
     d. Perineal or low back pain
     e. ARTHRALGIA

      f. Frequent, urgent urination

      g. Cloudy urine

      h. Dysuria

      i. Nocturia

      j. Urethral discharge

      k. On rectal palpation, prostate is tender, abnormally hard, swollen, and warm

  2. Chronic prostatitis

      a. May be symptom-free

      b. Frequent, urgent urination; perineal discomfort, low back pain

      c. Urethral discharge and painful ejaculation

      d. On rectal palpation, prostate may feel soft, and CREPITATION may be evident if prostatic calculi are present

  3. Nonbacterial prostatitis

      a. Dysuria

      b. Pain in penis, testes, scrotum, or lower back

      c. Nocturia

      d. Pain on ejaculation

      e. Prostate gland feels normal on palpation

      f. Decreased libido and impotence

C. Interventions

  1. Administer prescribed medications

      a. Systemic antibiotics (co-trimoxazole, minocycline, erythromycin, carbenicillin)

      b. Anticholinergics

      c. Analgesics

      d. Alpha-adrenergic blockers and muscle relaxants

      e. Stool softeners

      f. Antipyretics

  2. Bed rest

  3. Adequate hydration

  4. Sitz baths

  5. Regular massage of the prostate gland

  6. Regular ejaculation

  7. Possible resection of prostate

♦ III. Epididymitis

A. Pathophysiology

  1. Infection of epididymis, testicles' cordlike excretory ducts, which serve for storage, transport, and maturation of spermatozoa

  2. Usually a complication of urinary tract infection caused by PYOGENIC bacteria (urethritis or prostatitis)

  3. Pyogenic organisms reach epididymis through the urethra and lumen of the vas deferens

TEACHING TIPS
Patient with prostatitis

Be sure to include the following topics in your teaching plan for the patient with prostatitis:
• Be sure to complete the prescribed course of antibiotics.
• Avoid coffee, tea, alcohol, chocolate, cola, and spices, because they exert diuretic action and increase prostatic secretions.
• Drink adequate amounts of fluids but avoid forcing fluids because this reduces the medication level in the urine.
• Notify the doctor if symptoms recur.
• Teach the patient how to take a Sitz bath.

    4. Rarely, secondary to distant infection that spreads through the lymphatics or bloodstream

B. Assessment
    1. Unilateral pain, extreme tenderness, and edema in the groin and scrotum
    2. Erythema
    3. Fever
    4. Malaise
    5. Characteristic duck waddle, an attempt to protect the groin and scrotum during walking
    6. Acute hydrocele
    7. Dysuria

C. Interventions
    1. Bed rest
    2. Elevate scrotum and support with towel rolls or adhesive strapping
    3. When patient is ambulatory, advise wearing an athletic supporter to help prevent pain
    4. Administer prescribed medications
      a. Broad-spectrum antibiotics
      b. Analgesics, antipyretics

CLINICAL ALERT

    5. Apply ice bag to affected area
    6. Watch closely for abscess formation (localized, hot, red, tender area)
    7. Be alert for signs and symptoms of infection extension into the testes
      a. High fever
      b. Chills
      c. Sudden testicular pain radiating to inguinal area
      d. Nausea and vomiting

8. Advise patient to avoid sexual activity or physical strain (for additional teaching tips, see *Patient with prostatitis)*

♦ IV. Benign prostatic HYPERPLASIA

A. Pathophysiology

1. Prostate gland enlarges enough to compress the urethra and cause urinary obstruction

2. Increased estrogen levels in aging men prompt androgen receptors in the prostate gland to increase, causing overgrowth of normal cells that begins around the urethra

3. Additional causes of prostate enlargement
   a. Tumors (benign or malignant)
   b. Arteriosclerosis
   c. Inflammation
   d. Metabolic or nutritional disturbances

4. Enlargement that blocks the urethra and displaces the bladder upward may block urine flow and cause urinary tract infection or calculi formation

5. Bladder muscles may thicken and a DIVERTICULUM may form in the bladder that retains urine after the bladder empties

B. Assessment

1. Decreased volume and force of urine stream

2. Interrupted urine stream

3. Urinary hesitancy causing straining and a feeling of incomplete voiding

4. Patient may report additional symptoms as obstruction increases
   a. Frequent urination with nocturia
   b. Dribbling
   c. Urine retention
   d. Incontinence
   e. Blood in the urine

5. On rectal examination, an enlarged prostate is palpable

C. Interventions

1. "Watch and wait" policy to observe for regression or progression of disease

2. Administer prescribed medications
   a. Antimicrobials
   b. Terazosin to improve urine flow
   c. Alpha-adrenergics
   d. Androgen blockers, such as finasteride, flutamide; finasteride reduces prostate size

3. Prostate massage

4. Sitz baths

   5. Short-term fluid restrictions to prevent bladder distention
   6. Surgery
      a. Transurethral prostatic resection
      b. Suprapubic or perineal prostatectomy
      c. Transurethral incision of prostate
      d. Transurethral ultrasound-guided laser-induced prostatectomy
      e. Balloon dilation of prostatic portion of the urethra
      f. Microwave hyperthermia
      g. High-intensity focused ultrasound
      h. Transurethral needle ablation
      i. Stents

POINTS TO REMEMBER

◆ Early detection of male reproductive disorders is the key to preventing chronic or possibly irreversible conditions, such as sexual function and reproductive ability.

◆ A thorough physical examination and assessment of signs and symptoms is essential in diagnosing male reproductive disorders.

◆ Watch for possible reproductive tract problems when caring for a patient with a urinary tract disorder, especially if it involves infection or trauma.

STUDY QUESTIONS

To evaluate your understanding of this chapter, answer the following questions in the space provided; then compare your responses with the correct answers in appendix B, page 293.

1. Which microorganism causes prostatitis in 80% of cases? _____

   _____

2. How will the prostate feel on palpation in the patient with suspected acute prostatitis? _____

   _____

3. Why do patients with epididymitis develop a characteristic waddle?

   _____

   _____

4. What might a localized, hot, tender area in the testes indicate in a patient with epididymitis? _____

_____

5. During assessment, which symptoms should the nurse be alert for that might indicate urinary obstruction in benign prostatic hyperplasia? _____

_____

CRITICAL THINKING AND APPLICATION EXERCISES

1. Develop a chart comparing acute and chronic prostatitis. Include assessment findings and interventions.

2. Prepare a drug card for co-trimoxazole.

3. Observe a transurethral prostatic resection. Prepare an oral presentation for your fellow classmates describing the procedure and patient care before, during, and after the procedure.

4. Prepare a patient education sheet for postoperative care following transurethral prostatic resection.

5. Follow a patient with a male reproductive disorder from admission through discharge. Develop a plan of care, including any needs for follow-up and patient teaching.

Female reproductive disorders

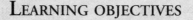

CHAPTER OVERVIEW

In many cases, female reproductive disorders occur simultaneously; for example, a patient with amenorrhea may also have an ovarian tumor, an infection, or a urologic disorder due to the proximity of the urinary and reproductive systems. A thorough assessment is necessary for diagnosis and prompt treatment. Interventions are geared to preserving childbearing abilities in females of childbearing age and preventing complications such as infertility.

◆ I. Types of disorders

A. Menstrual disorders
  1. May be primary, arising without any other disease state present
  2. May be secondary, indicating some other pathophysiologic process
  3. Most are related to a hormonal imbalance

B. Infections
  1. May result from sexually transmitted diseases (STDs), systemic infections, or organisms ascending from the lower to the upper urinary tract
  2. May lead to ectopic pregnancy or infertility

C. Benign tumors
  1. May affect the ovaries, uterus, or endometrium
  2. May produce no symptoms and may not cause debilitation

D. Cancer
  1. Malignant tumors can occur in every part of the female reproductive system
  2. Ovarian cancer is highly malignant; diagnosis is usually made only after metastasis has occurred (see chapter 19 for more information about ovarian cancer)

E. Breast disorders
  1. Disorders include fibrocystic changes and benign and malignant tumors
  2. Benign tumors can change with the menstrual cycle.
  3. Malignant tumors occur in epithelium of breast ducts and spread to lymph nodes (see chapter 19 for more information about breast cancer)

◆ II. Premenstrual syndrome

A. Pathophysiology
  1. Characterized by varying physical and psychological symptoms that appear 3 to 14 days before menses and usually subside with its onset
  2. Possible causes
     a. Endocrine imbalances (such as hyperprolactinemia, estrogen excess, altered estrogen-progesterone ratio, aldosterone excess)
     b. Altered endorphin activity
     c. Pyridoxine deficiency
  3. Influenced by learned beliefs about menstruation; for example, periods are expected to be painful and debilitating

B. Assessment
  1. Behavioral signs and symptoms
     a. Mild to severe personality changes
     b. Nervousness, anxiety

     c. Hostility

     d. Irritability

     e. Agitation

     f. Sleep disturbances

     g. Fatigue

     h. Lethargy

     i. Depression

  2. Somatic signs and symptoms

     a. Breast tenderness or swelling

     b. Abdominal tenderness, pain, or bloating

     c. Joint pain

     d. Headache, backache

     e. Edema, weight gain

     f. Diarrhea or constipation

     g. Worsening skin problems (such as acne or rashes)

     h. Worsening respiratory problems (such as asthma)

     i. Worsening neurologic problems (such as seizures)

C. Interventions

  1. Recommend a diet low in simple sugars, caffeine, and salt; high in lean protein

  2. Administer prescribed medications

     a. Diuretics

     b. Antidepressants, tranquilizers

     c. Vitamin and mineral supplements, such as B complex, vitamin E, and magnesium

     d. Hormonal supplement, replacement, or inhibitors dependent on underlying endocrine finding

     e. Prostaglandin inhibitors

     f. Nonsteroidal anti-inflammatory drugs (NSAIDs), mild analgesics

  3. Encourage regular exercise; relaxation techniques; lifestyle changes as appropriate

◆ III. Toxic shock syndrome

A. Pathophysiology

  1. An acute bacterial infection caused by toxin-producing, penicillin-resistant strains of *Staphylococcus aureus*

  2. When not related to menstruation, it may be linked to *S. aureus* infections such as abscesses, osteomyelitis, postsurgical infections, and childbirth or abortion

  3. Shock state can progress to severe hypotension, adult respiratory distress syndrome, and disseminated intravascular coagulation

  4. Primarily affects menstruating women under age 30

  5. Associated with continuous use of tampons during the menstrual period

B. Assessment
1. Intense myalgias
2. Fever over 104° F (40° C)
3. Headache
4. Decreased level of consciousness; dizziness, confusion, disorientation without focal signs
5. RIGORS
6. Conjunctival HYPEREMIA
7. Vaginal hyperemia and discharge
8. Severe hypotension
9. Deep red rash, especially on palms and soles
10. Sore throat
11. Vomiting; watery diarrhea

C. Interventions
1. Monitor vital signs frequently
2. Administer I.V. antibiotics, as ordered
3. Replace fluids with saline solution and colloids, as ordered
4. Monitor fluid and electrolytes
5. Tell patient to avoid superabsorbent tampons.

♦ IV. Pelvic inflammatory disease

A. Pathophysiology
1. Any acute, subacute, recurrent, or chronic polymicrobial infection of the oviducts and ovaries; may also involve the cervix, uterus, fallopian tubes, or connective tissue lying between the broad ligaments
2. Can result from infection by aerobic or anaerobic organisms; commonly (80%) due to *Neisseria gonorrhoeae* and *Chlamydia trachomatis*
   a. Conditions or procedures may alter or destroy bacteriostatic cervical mucus, allowing bacteria present in the cervix or vagina to ascend into the uterine cavity
   b. Infection can follow transfer of contaminated cervical mucus into the endometrial cavity by instrumentation
   c. Bacteria may enter the uterine cavity through the bloodstream
   d. Bacteria may enter from other infectious foci such as lymphatics
3. Risk factors
   a. Ages 16 to 24
   b. Nulliparity
   c. History of multiple sexual partners
   d. Previous history of PID
4. Complications include ectopic pregnancy, sterility, adhesions, and abscesses

B. Assessment
1. Profuse, purulent vaginal discharge

2. Fever
3. Malaise
4. Lower abdominal pain
5. Movement of the cervix or palpation of the adnexa may be extremely painful

C. Interventions
1. Administer prescribed medications
   a. Antibiotics (follow Centers for Disease Control and Prevention's STD guidelines)
   b. Analgesics, antipyretics
2. Monitor vital signs and fluid intake and output
3. Drainage of abscesses

CLINICAL
ALERT

4. Surgery if abscess ruptures
5. Watch for abdominal rigidity and distention, possible signs of developing peritonitis
6. To prevent a recurrence, explain the nature and seriousness of PID and encourage the patient to comply with the treatment regimen (for additional teaching tips, see *Patient with pelvic inflammatory disease*)

♦ V. Endometriosis

A. Pathophysiology
1. Presence of endometrial tissue outside the lining of the uterine cavity (ectopic)
2. Ectopic tissue most commonly develops around the ovaries (chocolate cysts), uterovesical peritoneum, uterosacral ligaments, cul-de-sac, pelvis, vagina, or intestines, but it may appear anywhere in the body
3. During menstruation the ectopic tissue bleeds, causing inflammation of the surrounding tissues
4. Inflammation leads to fibrosis, with adhesions that can produce pain, infertility, and bowel obstruction
5. Cause unknown; several risk factors
   a. Delayed childbearing
   b. Early menarche
   c. Regular periods with shorter cycles, longer duration, and heavier flow
   d. First-degree relatives with the disorder

B. Assessment
1. Classic triad includes dysmenorrhea (may produce pain in the lower abdomen, the vagina, posterior pelvis, and back), dyspareunia, and infertility
2. Pain begins 5 to 7 days before menses and lasts for 2 to 3 days

3. Other clinical findings depend on the location of the ectopic tissue
   a. Ovaries and oviducts: infertility and profuse menses
   b. Ovaries or cul-de-sac: deep-thrust dyspareunia
   c. Bladder: suprapubic pain, dysuria, hematuria
   d. Small bowel and appendix: nausea and vomiting (worsens before menses), abdominal cramps
   e. Cervix, vagina, and perineum: bleeding from endometrial deposits in these areas during menses

C. Interventions
   1. Administer prescribed medications
      a. Pain relief (NSAIDs)
      b. Endometrial suppression
         (1) Progesterone
         (2) Oral contraceptives
         (3) Androgens
         (4) Gonadotropin-releasing hormone antagonists
   2. Surgery
      a. Laparoscopy (laser surgery) to remove endometrial implants
      b. Total abdominal hysterectomy with bilateral salpingo-oophorectomy
      c. Pregnancy commonly results in atrophy of endometrial tissue

◆ VI. Fibrocystic breast changes

A. Pathophysiology
   1. One or more palpable cysts develop in the breast
   2. Usually causes one or both breasts to become lumpy and tender approximately 1 week before menses begins
   3. May be related to a hormonal imbalance
   4. Some fibrocystic tissues undergo malignant changes

TEACHING TIPS
Patient with fibrocystic breast changes

Be sure to include the following topics in your teaching plan for the patient with fibrocystic breast disease:
- Encourage use of a supportive bra.
- Instruct the patient to reduce intake of caffeine and salt, especially premenstrually.
- Avoid sleeping in prone position.
- Take steps to avoid or limit stress.
- Join in a planned exercise and activity program.

   B. Assessment
     1. Palpation of one or more lumps
     2. Tenderness or pain of the breast

   C. Interventions
     1. Apply local heat or cold
     2. Administer prescribed analgesics
     3. Drainage of fibrocystic lumps
     4. Surgical removal of lumps
     5. Danocrine (antiestrogenic effect) for severe cases
     6. Teach patient to perform monthly breast self-examination (for additional teaching tips, see *Patient with fibrocystic breast changes*)
     7. Give vitamin A, E, or B complex to relieve fluid engorgement

POINTS TO REMEMBER

◆ Infections must be treated promptly to prevent possible infertility.

◆ A thorough assessment is necessary to accurately diagnose some female reproductive disorders.

◆ Malignant tumors can be found in every part of the female reproductive system.

STUDY QUESTIONS

To evaluate your understanding of this chapter, answer the following questions in the space provided; then compare your responses with the correct answers in appendix B, page 293.

1. Which type of diet should a patient with PMS follow? _____

_____

2. What would abdominal rigidity and distention be signs of in the patient with PID? _____

_____

3. When during the menstrual cycle does the pain of endometriosis usually begin? _____

_____

4. Which medications are used to treat endometriosis? _____

_____

5. Which nursing intervention is important to teach to patients with fibrocystic breast changes? _____

_____

CRITICAL THINKING AND APPLICATION EXERCISES

1. Prepare a patient education sheet for hormone replacement therapy.

2. Prepare a presentation for your classmates on teaching breast self-examination.

3. Interview several patients with PMS about how it affects their lives. Present your information to your classmates for discussion about how to address the patient's issues.

4. Follow a patient with a female reproductive disorder from admission through discharge. Develop a patient-specific plan of care, including any need for follow-up and patient teaching.

Sexually transmitted diseases

LEARNING OBJECTIVES

After studying this chapter, you should be able to:

♦ Identify which tissues are susceptible to chlamydial infection.

♦ Discuss symptoms of chlamydial infection.

♦ Identify which virus causes condylomata acuminata.

♦ Discuss the stages of syphilis.

♦ Develop a plan of care according to the stage of syphilis.

♦ Assess and plan care for a patient with a sexually transmitted disease (STD).

♦ List STDs that are reportable to public health agencies.

♦ Discuss patient education for STDs.

CHAPTER OVERVIEW

Many sex-related disorders result from infection that is transmitted through sexual contact. STDs can show mild, severe, or no symptoms. A thorough assessment is necessary for effective treatment. Interventions aim to cure the disease with medication, relieve symptoms where there is no cure, and help prevent the spread of STDs through public health agencies and patient education.

♦ I. Pathophysiologic processes

A. Some STDs involve genitourinary organs
   1. In men: Urethritis, prostatitis, or epididymitis (for more about prostatitis and epididymitis, see chapter 13)
   2. In women: Urethritis, pelvic inflammatory disease (PID), or cervicitis (for more about PID, see chapter 14)

B. Some types of STDs, such as gonorrhea and syphilis, are systemic as well, starting in genitourinary organs and sometimes progressing to involve the heart or the central nervous system, or both

♦ II. Chlamydia

A. Pathophysiology
   1. A group of infections that are linked to one organism, *Chlamydia trachomatis*
   2. Transmission of *C. trachomatis* primarily follows vaginal or rectal intercourse or orogenital contact with an infected person; incubation period is 2 weeks
   3. Neonates of mothers who have chlamydial infections may contract associated conjunctivitis, otitis media, or pneumonia during passage through the birth canal
   4. Urethritis is a common infection in men; chlamydial infection may ascend to produce epididymitis or prostatitis
      a. Reiter's syndrome (urethritis, conjunctivitis, arthritis, and mucocutaneous lesions) may develop
      b. Syndrome is a type of reactive arthritis due to infection elsewhere in the body (usually genitourinary or enteric)
   5. In women, cervicitis is a common infection; chlamydial infection may ascend to produce salpingitis or endometritis (PID)

B. Assessment
   1. May be asymptomatic
   2. Signs and symptoms vary with the specific type of chlamydial infection and are determined by the organism's route of transmission to susceptible tissue
      a. Cervicitis: cervical erosion, mucopurulent discharge, pelvic pain, and dyspareunia
      b. Endometritis or salpingitis: pain and tenderness of the abdomen, cervix, uterus, and lymph nodes; chills; fever; breakthrough bleeding after intercourse; and vaginal discharge
      c. Urethral syndrome: dysuria, pyuria, and urinary frequency
      d. Male urethritis: dysuria, tenderness of urinary meatus, erythema, urinary frequency, pruritus, and urethral discharge
      e. Epididymitis: painful scrotal swelling and urethral discharge

     f. Prostatitis: low back pain, urinary frequency, dysuria, nocturia, and painful ejaculations

     g. Proctitis: diarrhea, TENESMUS, pruritus, bloody or mucopurulent discharge, diffuse or discrete ulceration in the rectosigmoid colon

C. Interventions

  1. Administer doxycycline or azithromycin, as prescribed

  2. If required in your state, report all cases of chlamydial infection to the appropriate local public health authorities

  3. Check newborns of infected mothers for signs of chlamydial infection

  4. Teach the patient to practice meticulous personal hygiene measures

  5. For additional teaching tips, see *Patient with chlamydia*

♦ III. Condylomata acuminata

A. Pathophysiology

  1. Also known as genital or venereal warts

  2. Infection with one of the more than 60 known strains of human papillomavirus (HPV) causes the warts, which are transmitted through sexual contact and enter the body through the mucous membranes

  3. Warts consist of PAPILLOMAS with fibrous tissue overgrowth from dermis and thickened epithelial coverings

  4. Warts grow rapidly in presence of heavy perspiration, poor hygiene, or pregnancy, and commonly accompany other genital infections

  5. Warts have a 1- to 8-month incubation period

  6. Uncommon before puberty and after menopause

  7. Certain types of HPV have been strongly associated with cervical intraepithelial neoplasia

B. Assessment

  1. Most patients report no symptoms

  2. Develops on moist body surfaces

     a. Males: on the subpreputial sac, within the urinary meatus, on the penile shaft

     b. Females: on the vulva, and on the vaginal and cervical walls

     c. Both sexes: papillomas spread to the perineum and the perianal area

  3. Appear as tiny red or pink swellings that grow (up to 4″ [10 cm]); may be papilliform, flat, or spiked

  4. If infected, these become malodorous

  5. Itching or pain in affected areas

C. Interventions

  1. Administer prescribed medications

     a. 10% to 25% podophyllum in tincture of benzoin

     b. Purified podophyllotoxin

TEACHING TIPS
Patient with chlamydia

Be sure to include the following topics in your teaching plan for the patient with chlamydia:
• Instruct the patient to avoid touching any discharge and to wash and dry hands thoroughly before touching the eyes.
• Advise the patient to prevent reinfection during treatment by abstaining from intercourse or using condoms until both partners are cured.
• Urge the patient to inform sexual contacts of the infection so that they can receive appropriate treatment.
• Ask the patient to consider being tested for human immunodeficiency virus (HIV) infection.

      c. Trichloroacetic acid
      d. Topical 5-fluorouracil
  2. For warts that are larger than 1″ (2.5 cm) in diameter
      a. Carbon dioxide laser treatment
      b. Cryosurgery
      c. Electrocautery
  3. Recommend abstinence from sexual intercourse or using a condom until healing is complete
  4. Encourage the patient's sexual partners to be examined for HPV, human immunodeficiency virus, and other sexually transmitted diseases
  5. Encourage annual Papanicolaou smears for women

♦ IV. Syphilis

A. Pathophysiology
  1. A chronic infectious, sexually transmitted disease caused by the spirochete *Treponema pallidum*
  2. Begins in the mucous membranes and quickly becomes systemic, spreading to nearby lymph nodes and the bloodstream
  3. When untreated, syphilis progresses through several stages: primary, secondary, latent, and tertiary
  4. Untreated syphilis leads to crippling and death
  5. Fetus can be infected by the mother transplacentally

B. Assessment
  1. Primary syphilis
      a. One or more CHANCRES erupt on the genitalia at the site of exposure; others may erupt on the anus, fingers, lips, tongue, nipples, tonsils, or eyelids

      b. Painless papules that erode to have indurated, raised edges and
         clear bases

      c. Disappear after 3 to 6 weeks

      d. Highly contagious

  2. Secondary syphilis

      a. Symmetrical mucocutaneous lesions and general lymphadenopa-
         thy

      b. Rash can be macular, papular, pustular, or nodular

      c. Macules often erupt on palms and soles, but they also commonly
         appear between rolls of fat on the trunk and proximally on the
         arms, face, and scalp

      d. Lesions on perineum, scrotum, vulva, between rolls of fat enlarge
         and erode, producing highly contagious, pink or grayish white
         lesions

      e. Headache

      f. Malaise

      g. Anorexia

      h. Weight loss

      i. Nausea and vomiting

      j. Sore throat, stomatitis

      k. Fever

      l. Alopecia

      m. Brittle, pitted nails

  3. Latent syphilis (asymptomatic)

  4. Tertiary syphilis (three forms)

      a. Late benign or gumma syphilis: lesions (gummas) develop on the
         skin, bones, mucous membranes, upper respiratory tract, testes,
         liver, or stomach

      b. Cardiovascular syphilis: aortitis with aortic insufficiency or
         aneurysm

      c. Neurosyphilis: meningitis, general paresis, personality changes,
         arm and leg weakness, ataxia and sensory loss (tabes dorsalis)

C. Interventions

  1. Administer penicillin; tetracycline or doxycycline if allergic to peni-
    cillin; erythromycin if pregnant

  2. Report all cases of syphilis to public health authorities

  3. Urge the patient to inform his sexual partners of his infection so
    that they can receive treatment

  4. In secondary syphilis, keep lesions clean and dry; if draining, dis-
    pose of contaminated materials properly

  5. In tertiary syphilis, provide asymptomatic care during prolonged
    treatment

6. In cardiovascular syphilis, check for signs of decreased cardiac output (decreased urine output, hypoxia, and decreased sensorium) and pulmonary congestion

7. In neurosyphilis, regularly check level of consciousness, mood, and coherence; watch for signs of ataxia

8. Urge patients to seek serologic testing after 3, 6, 12, and 24 months, to detect possible relapse

POINTS TO REMEMBER

♦ Early detection of STDs is the key to preventing complications.

♦ A thorough assessment of symptoms is essential in diagnosing and treating sexually transmitted diseases.

♦ The full course of antibiotic therapy must be completed even after symptoms subside.

STUDY QUESTIONS

To evaluate your understanding of this chapter, answer the following questions in the space provided; then compare your responses with the correct answers in appendix B, page 293.

1. What is the incubation period in *Chlamydia?* _____

_____

2. Which medications are routinely given to treat *Chlamydia?*_____

_____

3. Which organism causes condylomata acuminata? _____

_____

4. Why is it important to encourage annual Papanicolaou tests for women with HPV? _____

_____

5. How often following treatment should patients seek serologic testing to detect possible relapse of syphilis? _____

_____

CRITICAL THINKING AND APPLICATION EXERCISES

1. Prepare drug cards for ceftriaxone and penicillin.

2. Prepare a patient education sheet for antibiotic therapy.

3. Develop a chart comparing the different stages of syphilis. Include assessment findings, treatment, and nursing interventions.

4. Research the support groups in your area for patients with STDs. Include national and local groups.

5. Research your state's legal requirements for reporting STDs.

6. Interview several patients with STDs about how it affects their lives. Present your information to your classmates for discussion about how to address the patients' issues.

7. Follow a patient with a STD from admission to discharge. Develop a patient-specific plan of care, including any needs for follow-up and patient teaching.

16

Eye, Ear, Nose, and Throat Disorders

LEARNING OBJECTIVES

After studying this chapter, you should be able to:

♦ List the probable causes of retinal detachment.

♦ Discuss postoperative nursing interventions following surgery for retinal detachment.

♦ Describe the two types of age-related macular degeneration.

♦ List assessment findings for the different types of glaucoma.

♦ Discuss acute and chronic otitis media.

♦ Describe the characteristic assessment findings in Ménière's disease.

♦ Discuss nursing interventions for sinusitis.

CHAPTER OVERVIEW

Disorders of the eye, ear, nose and throat (EENT) require a thorough examination to determine diagnosis and plan nursing interventions. Interventions are geared to controlling and correcting the problem, promoting normal function, and preventing complications.

♦ I. Classes of disorders

A. Disorders of the *structures* of the EENT
1. Cause change in an organ's structure
2. May or may not affect organ's function
3. Include retinal detachment and cataracts

B. Disorders of the *function* of the EENT
1. Affect the function of these organs
2. Include infections such as otitis media, sinusitis, and tonsillitis

♦ II. Retinal detachment

A. Pathophysiology
1. Layers of the retina become separated, creating a subretinal space and disrupting retinal blood supply
2. Space then fills with fluid called subretinal fluid
3. In adults, usually results from degenerative changes of aging, which causes spontaneous holes to develop
4. Predisposing factors include myopia, cataract surgery, trauma
5. May also be caused by seepage of fluid into retinal space due to other conditions such as inflammation, tumors, systemic diseases, or congenital abnormalities
6. Detachment may also result from traction placed on retina by vitreous bands or membranes due to diabetic retinopathy, posterior uveitis, or a traumatic intraocular foreign body
7. Rarely occurs in children; may develop from retinopathy due to prematurity, tumors (such as retinoblastomas), or trauma

B. Assessment
1. Patient may complain of floaters, PHOTOPSIA ("flashing lights"), and photophobia
2. As detachment progresses, gradual, painless vision loss may be described as a veil, curtain, or cobweb that eliminates a portion of the visual field

C. Interventions
1. Treatment depends on location and severity of the detachment
2. Restriction of eye movements (eye patching) and complete bed rest to prevent further detachment
3. Cryotherapy to treat a hole in the peripheral retina
4. Laser therapy
5. Scleral buckling or pneumatic retinopathy may be required to reattach retina
6. Possible replacement of the vitreous with silicone, oil, air, or gas
7. Provide emotional support
8. Administer antibiotics and cycloplegic-mydriatic eyedrops, as prescribed

TEACHING TIPS
Patient with retinal detachment

Be sure to include the following topics in your teaching plan for the patient with retinal detachment:
• Instruct the patient to lie on his back or on his unoperated side.
• Discourage straining at stool, bending down, hard coughing, sneezing, and vomiting, which can raise intraocular pressure.
• Discourage activities that may cause the patient to bump his eye.
• Teach how to instill eyedrops.
• Suggest dark glasses to compensate for light sensitivity.

9. Teach the patient about appropriate postoperative care (for additional teaching tips, see *Patient with retinal detachment*)
10. To reduce edema and discomfort, apply ice packs, as ordered
11. Administer acetaminophen, as ordered, for headache and cycloplegic eyedrops and steroid-antibiotic eyedrops as prescribed.

♦ III. Age-related macular degeneration

A. Pathophysiology
1. Results from hardening and obstruction of retinal arteries that probably reflect normal degenerative changes; characterized by loss of central vision (usually bilateral); cause unknown
2. Disorder occurs in two forms
   a. Dry (atrophic) form, marked by atrophic degeneration of photoreceptors, causes slow, progressive visual loss
   b. Wet (exudative) form, marked by subretinal neovascularization that causes leakage, hemorrhage, and fibrovascular scarring, causes significant loss of central vision
3. Underlying pathologic changes occur primarily in retinal pigment, epithelium, Bruch's membrane, and lamina choroidocapillaris in the macular region

B. Assessment
1. Changes in central vision; blank spot appears in the center of the page when reading
2. Difficulty with seeing near or far, differentiating colors, recognizing faces
3. Appearance of drusen (pale, yellow spots or bumps) on macula

C. Interventions
1. Dry atrophic form: no successful treatment; low-vision optical aids may be helpful
2. Wet, exudative form: laser photocoagulation

3. Inform patients with bilateral central loss about visual rehabilitation services available to them

♦ IV. Cataract

A. Pathophysiology

1. A gradually developing opacity of the lens or lens capsule
2. Commonly occurs bilaterally and may progress independently except in some conditions, such as traumatic cataracts (unilateral) and congenital cataracts (may remain stationary)
3. Various types of cataracts are known
   a. Senile: develop in elderly from degenerative changes in the chemical state of lens proteins
   b. Congenital: occur in newborns as genetic defects or as a sequela of maternal rubella during first trimester
   c. Traumatic: develop after a foreign body or blunt trauma injures the lens with enough force to allow aqueous or vitreous humor to enter lens capsule
   d. Complicated: develop as secondary effects in patients with uveitis, glaucoma, retinitis pigmentosa, or detached retina; or accompany systemic disorder of carbohydrate metabolism (such as diabetes mellitus)
   e. Toxic: from toxic reactions to drugs or chemicals such as corticosteroids, ergot alkaloids, dinitrophenol, naphthalene, phenothiazines, busulfan, or pilocarpine; or secondary to ultraviolet exposure

B. Assessment

1. Painless, gradual blurring and visual distortion
2. Normally black pupil turns milky white
3. Complaints of blinding glare from headlights when driving at night
4. Complaints of poor reading vision
5. Unpleasant glare and poor vision in bright sunlight
6. Problems with far and near vision

C. Interventions

1. Several surgical approaches
   a. Extracapsular cataract extraction and posterior chamber intraocular lens implant
   b. Phacoemulsification
   c. Intracapsular cataract extraction
   d. Discission and aspiration (now rarely used)
   e. YAG (yttrium-aluminum-garnet) laser
2. Postoperative care
   a. Remind the patient to return for a checkup the day following surgery
   b. Warn patients to avoid activities that increase intraocular pressure, such as straining, bending, coughing

    c. Urge the patient to protect the eye from accidental injury by wearing an eye shield or glasses during the day and an eye shield at night

    d. Administer cycloplegic-mydriatic eyedrops and antibiotic ointment or drops

    e. Watch for complications such as prolapsed iris, sharp pain in the eye, or HYPHEMA

    f. Teach correct instillation of eyedrops

    g. Inform patient that it will take several weeks before he will receive corrective reading glasses or lenses

♦ V. Glaucoma

A. Pathophysiology

    1. A group of disorders marked by abnormally high intraocular pressure (IOP), which can damage the optic nerve

    2. Untreated disease leads to gradual vision loss and blindness

    3. Several forms of glaucoma

      a. Open-angle: results from overproduction of aqueous humor or obstruction to its outflow through the trabecular network or the canal of Schlemm, causing consistently elevated IOP

      b. Acute angle-closure: closure results from obstructed outflow of aqueous humor due to anatomically narrow angles between the anterior iris and the posterior corneal surface; shallow anterior chambers; a thickened iris that causes angle closure on pupil dilation; or a bulging iris

      c. Secondary: results from inflammatory problems in the eyes, from tumors, or from extravasated red blood cells that obstruct outflow of aqueous humor

B. Assessment

    1. Open-angle glaucoma

      a. Usually bilateral with insidious onset

      b. Mild aching in the eye

      c. Loss of peripheral vision (tunnel vision); blurred vision

      d. Seeing halos around lights

      e. Reduced visual acuity not correctable with glasses

      f. Cupping of optic discs

    2. Acute angle-closure glaucoma

      a. Rapid onset; can lead to blindness in 3 to 5 days

      b. Unilateral inflammation and pain

      c. Pressure over the eye

      d. Moderate pupil dilation that is nonreactive to light

      e. Cloudy cornea

      f. Blurring and decreased visual acuity

      g. Photophobia

h. Seeing halos around lights

i. Nausea, vomiting

C. Interventions

1. Administer prescribed medications

a. Beta blockers, such as timolol

b. Prostaglandin analogues

b. Epinephrine

c. Diuretics

d. Miotic eyedrops

2. Surgical procedures

a. Argon laser trabeculoplasty

b. Trabeculectomy

c. Peripheral iridectomy/iridotomy

◆ VI. Otitis media

A. Pathophysiology

1. Results from disruption of eustachian tube patency resulting in accumulation of fluid in middle ear

2. Inflammation of the middle ear, may be suppurative or serous, acute or chronic

3. Acute form common in children

4. Prolonged accumulation of fluid in the middle ear cavity causes chronic otitis media and possibly perforation of the tympanic membrane

5. In the *suppurative* form, respiratory tract infection, allergic reactions, nasotracheal intubation, or positional changes allow nasopharyngeal flora to reflux through the eustachian tube and proliferate in the middle ear

6. In the *serous* form, an obstruction of the eustachian tube causes a buildup of negative pressure in the middle ear that promotes transudation of sterile serous fluid from blood vessels in the membrane of the middle ear

7. Chronic serous otitis media follows persistent eustachian tube dysfunction from mechanical obstruction, edema, or inadequate treatment of acute suppurative otitis media

B. Assessment

1. Acute suppurative otitis media

a. Severe, deep throbbing pain

b. Signs of upper respiratory infection

c. Mild to very high fever

d. Hearing loss

e. Tinnitus

f. Dizziness

g. Nausea and vomiting

TEACHING TIPS
Patient with otitis media

Be sure to include the following topics in your teaching plan for the patient with otitis media:
• Complete full course of prescribed antibiotics.
• Avoid getting water in ears; use ear plugs as needed.
• Seek prompt treatment of upper respiratory infection.
• Avoid cleaning ears with small hard objects such as cotton swabs, bobby pins, or matchsticks.

---

       h. Bulging of tympanic membrane, with concomitant erythema
       i. Purulent drainage in ear canal from tympanic membrane rupture
   2. Acute serous otitis media
       a. Severe conductive hearing loss
       b. Sensation of fullness in the ear
       c. Popping, crackling, or clicking sounds on swallowing or with jaw movements
   3. Chronic otitis media
       a. Thickening and scarring of the tympanic membrane
       b. Decreased or absent tympanic membrane mobility
       c. CHOLESTEATOMA
       d. Painless, purulent drainage

C. Interventions
   1. Administer prescribed medications
       a. Antibiotics
       b. Analgesics
       c. Antipyretics
       d. Nasal decongestants, antihistamines (controversial)
   2. Teach patient about avoiding allergens, as appropriate (for additional teaching tips, see *Patient with otitis media*)
   3. Apply local heat
   4. Perform myringotomy postoperative care
       a. Don't place cotton or plugs deep in the ear canal; sterile cotton may be placed loosely in the external ear canal to absorb drainage
       b. Change the cotton whenever it gets damp
       c. Monitor for headache, fever, severe pain, or disorientation
       d. Position patient on affected side to facilitate drainage
   5. Perform tympanoplasty postoperative care
       a. Reinforce dressings and observe for excessive bleeding from the ear canal
       b. Warn patient against blowing his nose or getting his ear wet when bathing

◆ VII. Ménière's disease

A. Pathophysiology

1. May result from overproduction or decreased absorption of endolymph
2. Endolymphatic hypertension ensues, causing degeneration of vestibular and cochlear hair cells
3. Disease may also stem from autonomic nervous system dysfunction that temporarily constricts blood vessels supplying the inner ear; may be secondary to viral injury
4. In some women, premenstrual edema may precipitate attacks of Ménière's disease

B. Assessment

1. Four characteristic effects
   a. Severe rotary vertigo
   b. Tinnitus
   c. Sensorineural hearing loss
   d. Feelings of fullness in the ear
2. Other signs and symptoms during acute attack
   a. Nausea and vomiting
   b. Sweating, pallor
   c. Giddiness
   d. Nystagmus
   e. Characteristic posture: lying on the unaffected ear and looking in the direction of the affected ear

C. Interventions

1. Administer prescribed medications
   a. Prochlorperazine, diazepam, promethazine
   b. Histamine analogues
   c. Diuretic or vasodilator for long-term management
   d. Corticosteroids
2. Low-sodium diet
3. Surgery
4. Chemical ablation with streptomycin

◆ VIII. Sinusitis

A. Pathophysiology

1. Inflammation of the paranasal sinuses; may be acute, subacute, chronic, allergic, or hyperplastic
2. Acute suppurative sinusitis usually results from the common cold and lingers in subacute form in only about 10% of patients
3. Chronic sinusitis follows persistent bacterial infection
4. Allergic sinusitis accompanies allergic rhinitis

5. Hyperplastic sinusitis results from bacterial growth on the diseased tissue, causing tissue edema and thickening of the mucosal lining as well as development of nasal polyps

B. Assessment
1. Acute sinusitis
   a. Nasal congestion
   b. Malaise
   c. Sore throat
   d. Headache, facial pain
   e. Low-grade fever
   f. Decreased sense of smell; purulent nasal discharge
   g. Characteristic pain depends on the affected sinus
2. Subacute sinusitis
   a. Purulent nasal drainage that continues from 3 weeks to 3 months after an acute infection
   b. Stuffy nose
   c. Vague facial discomfort
   d. Fatigue
   e. Nonproductive cough
3. Chronic sinusitis
   a. Similar to acute, but there is continuous mucopurulent discharge
   b. Loss of smell
   c. Postnasal drip
   d. Chronic cough
4. Allergic sinusitis
   a. Sneezing
   b. Frontal headache
   c. Watery, nasal discharge
   d. Stuffy, burning, itchy nose
5. Hyperplastic sinusitis
   a. Chronic stuffiness of the nose
   b. Headaches

C. Interventions
1. Administer prescribed medications
   a. Decongestants; antihistamines (controversial)
   b. Antibiotics
   c. Steroid or saline nasal spray
   d. Analgesics
   e. Expectorants
2. Apply warm compresses; steam inhalation
3. Irrigation of the sinuses
4. Endoscopic sinus surgery: partial or total resection of the middle turbinates; total sphenoethmoidectomy

5. Postoperative care
   a. Tell patient to expect nasal packing after surgery
   b. Monitor for excessive drainage or bleeding
   c. To prevent edema and promote drainage, place patient in semi-Fowler's position
   d. Apply ice compresses over nose and iced saline gauze over the eyes for first 24 hours
   e. Because patient will be breathing through his mouth, provide meticulous mouth care

POINTS TO REMEMBER

♦ A thorough assessment is essential in making a diagnosis.

♦ Treatment and interventions should begin promptly to prevent complications and prevent further deterioration of vision or hearing.

STUDY QUESTIONS

To evaluate your understanding of this chapter, answer the following questions in the space provided; then compare your responses with the correct answers in appendix B, pages 293 and 294.

1. What are the two types of age-related macular degeneration? _____

    _____

2. How long will it take for blindness to develop in acute angle-closure glaucoma, if left untreated? _____

    _____

3. After a myringotomy, how should the nurse position the patient? _____

    _____

4. What are the four characteristic assessment findings in Ménière's disease?

    _____

    _____

5. Which type of sinusitis causes continuous mucopurulent nasal drainage?

    _____

    _____

CRITICAL THINKING AND APPLICATION EXERCISES

1. Prepare a patient education sheet on eyedrop instillation.

2. Prepare drug cards on the following: tetracycline, erythromycin, and sulfonamides.

3. Research visual rehabilitative services including local and national agencies.

4. Observe a tonsillectomy for a pediatric patient. Prepare an oral presentation for your fellow classmates describing the procedure and patient care before, during, and after the procedure.

5. Follow a patient with an EENT disorder from admission through discharge. Develop a patient-specific plan of care, including any needs for follow-up and patient teaching.

Skin Disorders

LEARNING OBJECTIVES

After studying this chapter, you should be able to:

♦ Discuss the various types of dermatitis, including assessment and interventions.

♦ Describe the pathophysiology of psoriasis.

♦ Describe the lesions and plaques of psoriasis.

♦ Discuss the mode of transmission of warts.

♦ List the assessment findings of the various kinds of warts.

♦ Describe the pathophysiology of acne vulgaris.

♦ Develop nursing interventions regarding acne vulgaris.

♦ Develop a plan of care for a patient with a skin disorder.

CHAPTER OVERVIEW

The skin is the body's first line of defense against infections, trauma, fluid loss, and many other environmental insults. Knowledge of the skin and its function provides the foundation for understanding the various disorders of the skin. Assessment and nursing interventions are geared to early diagnosis and treatment of these disorders.

◆ I. Introduction

A. General information
1. Skin is vulnerable to infection by parasites, bacteria, and viruses
2. It may also be affected by inflammation and other conditions related to genetic, hormonal, or immune disorders

B. Parasitic disorders
1. Parasites, such as the scabies mite, live and breed in skin tissue
2. If skin integrity is breached, inflammation and infection may result
3. Can occur in anyone at any time

C. Inflammatory disorders
1. Dermatitis can be caused by bacterial, viral, or fungal infection
2. May also result from an allergen, stress, or another disease

D. Hereditary or immune disorders
1. Psoriasis has unknown cause
2. May be caused by genetic, immune, and environmental factors

E. Infectious disorders
1. Warts caused by papillomaviruses
2. Growths are benign; in later years, body develops immunity to them

F. Hormonal disorders
1. Acne is caused by many factors
2. Excessive androgen secretion or related hormonal dysfunction sets the stage for development of skin problems

◆ II. Dermatitis

A. Pathophysiology
1. Inflammation of the skin occurs in several forms (see *Types of dermatitis*, pages 248 to 250)
2. Characterized by raised, scaling lesions

B. Assessment
1. Atopic
   a. Pruritis
   b. Edema
   c. Crusting and scaling
   d. Chronic atopic lesions lead to multiple areas of dry, scaly skin with white dermatographism, blanching, and lichenification
2. Common secondary conditions include viral, fungal, and bacterial infections, and ocular disorders

C. Interventions
1. Eliminate allergens
2. Avoid irritants, such as wool and lanolin

(Text continues on page 251.)

Types of dermatitis

TYPE	CAUSES	SIGNS AND SYMPTOMS	TREATMENT AND INTERVENTIONS
Seborrheic dermatitis An acute or subacute skin disease that affects the scalp, face and, occasionally, other areas and is characterized by lesions covered with yellow or brownish gray scales	• Unknown; stress and neurologic conditions may be predisposing factors, may be related to the yeast *Pityrosporum ovale*	• Eruptions in areas with many sebaceous glands (usually scalp, face, and trunk) and in skin folds • Itching, redness, and inflammations may appear greasy; fissures may occur • Indistinct, occasionally yellowish, scaly patches from excess stratum corneum (dandruff may be a mild seborrheic dermatitis) • Generally worse in winter	• Removal of scales with frequent washing and shampooing with selenium sulfide suspension (most effective), or zinc pyrithione • Application of fluorinated corticosteroids to nonhairy areas
Nummular dermatitis Chronic form of dermatitis characterized by inflammation of coin-shaped, vesicular, crusted scales and, possibly, pruritic lesions	• Possibly precipitated by stress, skin dryness, irritants, scratching, or bathing with hot water	• Round, nummular (coin-shaped) lesions; usually on arms and legs with distinct borders of crusts and scales • Possible oozing and severe itching • Summertime remissions common, with wintertime recurrence	• Elimination of known irritants • Measures to relieve dry skin; increased humidification; limited frequency of baths; use of bland soaps and bath oils, and application of emollients • Application of wet dressings in acute phase • Topical corticosteroids (occlusive dressings or intralesional injections) for persistent lesions •Antihistamines to control itching • Antibiotics for secondary infection • Other interventions as for atopic dermatitis
Contact dermatitis In many cases, sharply demarcated inflammation and irritation of the skin due to	• Mild irritants: chronic exposure to detergents or solvents	• Mild irritants and allergens: erythema and small vesicles that ooze, scale, and itch	• Elimination of known allergens and decreased exposure to irritants; wearing protective clothing such as gloves; and immediately washing after contact with allergens or irritants

Types of dermatitis (continued)

TYPE	CAUSES	SIGNS AND SYMPTOMS	TREATMENT AND INTERVENTIONS
Contact dermatitis *(continued)* contact with concentrated substances (irritants or allergens) to which the skin is sensitive, such as perfumes, soaps, chemicals, and poison ivy	• Strong irritants: damage on contact with acids or alkalies • Allergens: sensitization after repeated exposure (type IV hypersensitivity reaction)	• Strong irritants: blisters and ulcerations • Classic allergic response clearly defined lesions, with straight lines following points of contact • Severe allergic reaction: marked edema of affected areas	• Topical anti-inflammatory agents (including corticosteroids), systemic corticosteroids for edema and bullae, antihistamines, and local applications of Burow's solution (for blisters) • Sensitization to topical medications may occur • Other interventions as for atopic dermatitis
Chronic dermatitis Characterized by inflammatory eruptions of the hands and feet	• Usually unknown but may result from progressive contact dermatitis • Secondary (possibly perpetuating) factors: trauma, infections, redistribution of normal flora, photosensitivity, and food sensitivity	• Thick, lichenified, single or multiple lesions on any part of the body (commonly on the hands) • Inflammation and scaling • Recurrence following long remissions	• Antibiotics for secondary infection • Avoidance of excessive washing and drying of hands and of accumulation of soaps and detergents under rings • Use of emollients with topical steroids • Other interventions as for contact dermatitis
Localized neurodermatitis (Lichen simplex chronicus, essential pruritis) Superficial inflammation of the skin characterized by itching and papular eruptions that appear on thickened, hyperpigmented skin	• Chronic scratching or rubbing of a primary lesion or insect bite, or other skin irritation	• Intense, sometimes continual scratching • Thick, sharp-bordered, possibly dry, scaly lesions with raised papules • Usually affects easily reached areas, such as ankles, lower legs, anogenital area, back of neck, and ears	• Scratching must stop; then lesions will disappear in about 2 weeks • Fixed dressing or Unna's boot to cover affected area • Topical corticosteroids under occlusion or by intralesional injection • Antihistamines and open wet dressings • Emollients • Inform patient about underlying cause

(continued)

Types of dermatitis (continued)

TYPE	CAUSES	SIGNS AND SYMPTOMS	TREATMENT AND INTERVENTIONS
Exfoliative dermatitis Severe, chronic skin inflammation characterized by redness and widespread erythema and scaling	• Usually, prexisting skin lesions progress to exfoliative stage, such as in contact dermatitis, drug reaction, lymphoma, or leukemia	• Generalized dermatitis, with acute loss of stratum corneum, and erythema and scaling • Sensation of tight skin • Hair loss • Possible fever, sensitivity to cold, shivering, gynecomastia, and lymphadenopathy	• Hospitalization, with protective isolation and hygienic measures to prevent secondary bacterial infection • Open wet dressings, with colloidal baths • Bland lotions over topical corticosteroids • Maintenance of constant environmental temperature to prevent chilling or overheating • Careful monitoring of renal and cardiac status • Systemic antibiotics and steroids • Other interventions as for atopic dermatitis
Stasis dermatitis Condition usually caused by impaired circulation and characterized by eczema of the legs with edema, hyperpigmentation, and persistent inflammation	• Secondary to peripheral vascular diseases affecting legs, such as recurrent thrombophlebitis and resultant chronic venous insufficiency; familial	• Varicosities and edema common, but obvious vascular insufficiency not always present • Usually affects the lower leg, just above the internal malleolus, or sites of trauma or irritation • Early signs: dusky red deposits of hemosiderin in skin, with itching and dimpling of subcutaneous tissue. Later signs: edema, redness, and scaling of large areas of legs • Possible fissures, crusts, and ulcers	• Measures to prevent venous stasis: avoidance of prolonged sitting or standing, use of support stockings, and weight reduction in obesity; elevation of legs • Corrective surgery for underlying cause • After ulcer develops, encourage rest periods, with legs elevated; open wet dressings; Unna's boot (zinc gelatin dressing provides continuous pressure to affected areas); and antibiotics for secondary infection after wound culture • Corticosteroid ointment

3. Avoid extreme temperature and humidity changes (use humidifier or air conditioner)
4. Apply topical corticosteroid ointment, as ordered
5. Apply moisturizing cream after bathing; use least amount of soap and water for bathing; avoid lanolin-based preparations
6. Apply fluorinated corticosteroid ointment
7. Administer antihistamines (chlorpheniramine)
8. Administer antibiotics as indicated for secondary infection
9. Inform patient that emotional stress can exacerbate atopic dermatitis

♦ III. Psoriasis

A. Pathophysiology
1. Chronic, recurrent disease marked by epidermal proliferation
2. Life cycle of a psoriatic skin cell is only 4 days, which doesn't allow time for the cells to mature (normal skin cells live 28 days)
3. The stratum corneum becomes erythematous, thick, and flaky, producing the cardinal manifestation of psoriasis
4. Flare-ups are usually related to specific systemic and environmental factors
5. Skin trauma is common precipitating factor; other factors are hereditary and immune related
6. Not contagious
7. Possible association between psoriasis and arthritis; 5% to 7% develop arthritic symptoms in fingers, toes, or sacroiliac joint

B. Assessment
1. Itching and occasional pain
2. Erythematous, dry, cracked, encrusted lesions
3. Plaques consist of characteristic silver scales that either flake off easily or can thicken, covering the lesion
4. Commonly occurs on scalp, elbows, and knees, but can occur anywhere

C. Interventions
1. Administer prescribed topical medications
   a. Steroid creams and ointments
   b. Emollients
   c. Keratolytic agents
   d. Anthralin
   e. Calcipotriene
2. Administer prescribed systemic treatments
   a. Phototherapy: exposure to ultraviolet light (UVB or natural sunlight)
   b. Methotrexate
   c. Retinoids
   d. Corticosteroids

What happens in acne

In acne vulgaris, hormonal, bacterial, and inflammatory responses in the skin interact to produce the disorder.
• Androgens stimulate sebaceous glands to produce large amounts of sebum.
• Bacteria secrete lipase, which interacts with sebum and forms free fatty acids.
• Inflammatory response occurs in the pilosebaceous unit.
• Hyperkeratinization occurs in the lining of the follicle.
• Distended follicle walls break and the sebum, lipid, fatty acids, and keratin enter the dermis.
• Foreign body response takes place: papule, pustule, nodule formation.
• Dermis heals.
• Rupture and inflammation occur.
• Scar forms.

      e. Cyclosporine
      f. Photochemotherapy (methoxsalen)
    3. Make sure the patient understands his prescribed therapy and teach correct application of medications
    4. Watch for adverse reactions to medications

♦ **IV. Warts**

  A. Pathophysiology
    1. Common, benign, viral infections of the skin and adjacent membranes; also known as verrucae
    2. Caused by infection with the human papillomavirus
    3. Mode of transmission is probably through direct contact, but AUTOINOCULATION is possible

  B. Assessment
    1. Common warts: rough, elevated, rounded surface
    2. Filiform warts: single, thin, threadlike projections; usually on eyelids, face, and neck
    3. Periungual warts: rough, irregularly shaped, elevated surface
    4. Flat warts: multiple groupings slightly raised with smooth, flat, or slightly rounded tops
    5. Plantar warts: slightly elevated or flat on soles of feet
    6. Digitate warts: fingerlike, horny projections arising from a pea-shaped base

  C. Interventions
    1. Electrodesiccation and curettage
    2. Cryotherapy
    3. Acid therapy

TEACHING TIPS
Patient with acne

Be sure to include the following topics in your teaching plan for the patient with acne:
• Emphasize the importance of meticulous hygiene.
• Keep hair off face; shampoo daily if necessary
• Identify predisposing factors that may be eliminated or modified; avoid mechanical trauma.
• Instruct the patient in the correct application of medications, including benzoyl peroxide preparations (alone or in combination with tretinoin); topical or systemic antibiotics; estrogen; and keratolytic agents (sulfur, salicylic acid, resorcinol).
• Inform the patient that most acne medications cause some drying and peeling.

---

    4. Carbon dioxide laser therapy
    5. Tretinoin gel
    6. Mild corticosteroid cream
    7. Salicylic acid or cimetidine paste
    8. Psychotherapy

♦ V. Acne vulgaris

A. Pathophysiology
    1. An inflammatory disease of the sebaceous follicles that primarily affects adolescents
    2. Androgens stimulate sebaceous gland growth and production of sebum, which is secreted into hair follicles that contain bacteria
    3. The bacteria secrete lipase, which produces free fatty acids, causing inflammation (papules, pustules) (see *What happens in acne*)

B. Assessment
    1. May appear as a whitehead or blackhead, most commonly seen on the face, chest, and back; local tenderness
    2. In severe forms, will see acne cysts or abscesses
    3. Chronic, recurring lesions produce scars

C. Interventions
    1. Patient education (for teaching tips, see *Patient with acne*)
    2. Surgery
    3. UV radiation
    4. Cryosurgery
    5. Provide emotional support

POINTS TO REMEMBER

- ◆ A thorough assessment is essential to determine diagnosis and treatment.
- ◆ Patient education regarding medication therapy is important to prevent adverse reactions and a delay in healing.

STUDY QUESTIONS

To evaluate your understanding of this chapter, answer the following questions in the space provided; then compare your responses with the correct answers in appendix B, page 294.

1. What are some factors that can exacerbate atopic dermatitis? _____
   _____

2. What are the characteristics of psoriatic plaques?_____
   _____

3. Which organism causes warts?_____
   _____

4. What is the mode of transmission of warts?_____
   _____

CRITICAL THINKING AND APPLICATION EXERCISES

1. Prepare a patient education sheet for Tretinoin.

2. Research ultraviolet light (UVB) therapy.

3. Prepare a patient education sheet for steroid creams and ointments.

4. Interview several patients with acne about how it affects their lives. Present your information to your fellow classmates for discussion about how to address the patients' issues.

5. Follow a patient with a skin disorder from admission through discharge. Develop a patient-specific plan of care, including any needs for follow-up and patient teaching.

Genetic Disorders

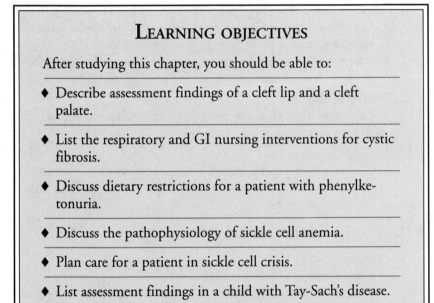

CHAPTER OVERVIEW

In this chapter you'll learn the about the pathophysiology, diagnostic tests, and interventions for several common genetic disorders. Nursing interventions are geared to supportive measures for the patient and parent of a child with a genetic disorder.

◆ I. Introduction

A. Chromosomes and genes
  1. Chromosomes contain deoxyribonucleic acid (DNA), which contains the genes
  2. Genes are the structures responsible for hereditary characteristics; they may or may not be expressed (passed to the next generation)
  3. Genetic disorders can be caused by chromosomal aberrations, a deviation in either the structure or the number of chromosomes
  4. Genetic disorders may be placed in two broad categories: single-gene disorders and sex-linked disorders

B. Single-gene disorders
  1. Autosomal dominant inheritance: only one parent needs to pass on a defective gene or set of genes to manifest disease
  2. Autosomal recessive inheritance: both parents must pass the defective gene or set of genes to the child to manifest disease

C. Sex-linked disorders
  1. Carried on the X chromosome and passed by women
  2. Women do not usually get these disorders

D. Multifactorial disorders
  1. Caused by both genetic and environmental factors
  2. Causes include maternal age, maternal infection, exposure to toxic chemicals (TERATOGENS)

◆ II. Cleft lip and cleft palate

A. Pathophysiology
  1. A multifactorial genetic disorder, cleft lip and cleft palate originate in the 2nd month of gestation, when the front and sides of the face and the shelves of the palate fuse imperfectly
  2. Four categories
    a. Clefts of the lip (unilateral or bilateral)
    b. Clefts of the palate (along the midline)
    c. Unilateral clefts of the lip, alveolar ridge, and palate
    d. Bilateral clefts of the lip, alveolar ridge, and palate

B. Assessment
  1. A cleft lip appears as anything from a simple notch to a complete cleft, and appears on either side of the nostril
  2. A cleft palate may be partial or complete, including the soft palate, the bones of the maxilla, and the alveolar ridge on one or both sides of the premaxilla

C. Interventions
  1. Prior to surgical correction

a. Maintain adequate nutrition by experimenting with feeding devices such as a nipple with a flange or regular nipple with enlarged holes

b. Begin to incorporate postoperative needs into the daily routine (for example, not lying in prone position, briefly applying arm restraints)

2. Surgical correction
   a. Cleft lip repaired shortly after birth
   b. Cleft palate repaired later (6 months to 1 year)

◆ III. Cystic fibrosis

A. Pathophysiology

1. A generalized dysfunction of the exocrine glands that affects multiple organ systems
2. Inherited as an autosomal recessive trait
3. Most cases arise from a mutation that affects the genetic coding for a single amino acid, resulting in a protein that doesn't function properly
4. The abnormal protein may interfere with chloride transport by preventing adenosine triphosphate from binding to the protein or by interfering with activation of protein kinase
5. The lack of an essential amino acid leads to dehydration and mucosal thickening in the respiratory and intestinal tracts

B. Assessment

1. Respiratory
   a. Frequent upper respiratory infections and pneumonia
   b. Dyspnea
   c. Paroxysmal cough
   d. Possible atelectasis or emphysema
2. GI
   a. Chronic pancreatitis
   b. Hepatic failure and cholecystitis may result from blockage of pancreatic ducts
   c. Deficiency of enzymes trypsin, amylase, and lipase may prevent the conversion and absorption of protein, carbohydrate, and fat in the intestinal tract; leads to malabsorption and steatorrhea
3. Reproductive
   a. Males may have lowered sperm counts
   b. Females may have secondary amenorrhea and increased mucus in the reproductive tract that blocks passage of the ovum

C. Interventions

1. Respiratory
   a. Administer antibiotics, as ordered
   b. Oxygen therapy and use of humidifiers and air conditioners

> **TEACHING TIPS**
> ## *Patient with cystic fibrosis*
>
> Be sure to include the following topics in your teaching plan for the patient with cystic fibrosis:
> • Advise the patient to consume a diet low in fat and high in protein and calories and to take vitamin supplements.
> • Teach parents about medications and treatments.
> • Contact resources, such as the Cystic Fibrosis Foundation, that provide help and support.
> • Teach parents or significant others how to perform chest physiotherapy.
> • Encourage genetic counseling for patients and families.

    c. Intermittent bronchodilator-nebulizer, chest physiotherapy, and postural drainage to loosen and remove secretions

    d. Recombinant DNAse, to thin mucous secretions

    e. Lung transplantation

  2. GI

    a. Give oral pancreatic enzymes with meals and snacks, as ordered, and salt replacement as needed

    b. Patient teaching (see *Patient with cystic fibrosis*)

◆ IV. Down syndrome

A. Pathophysiology

  1. Also called trisomy 21, Down syndrome is caused by an aberration in which chromosome 21 has three copies instead of the normal two because of nondisjunction (faulty meiosis) of the ovum

  2. In some cases, it is thought that the abnormality results from deterioration of the oocyte caused by age or cumulative effects of environmental factors

  3. Patients exhibit a karyotype of 47 chromosomes instead of the normal 46

  4. Increased prevalence in women age 35 or older

B. Assessment

  1. Physical signs apparent at birth

  2. Marked by craniofacial anomalies

    a. Slanting, almond-shaped eyes

    b. Protruding tongue

    c. Small, open mouth

    d. Small white spots on the iris

    e. Small skull

    f. Flattened bridge of nose

    g. Flattened face

h. Small, low-set, malformed ears
i. Short neck with excess skin
3. Additional findings
   a. Dry, sensitive skin with decreased elasticity
   b. Short stature with short extremities
   c. Hands and feet appear short, broad, flat and squarish, with wide space between the first and second toe
   d. Single, transverse crease on palm
   e. Decreased muscle tone in limbs impair reflex development
   f. Congenital heart disease
   g. Duodenal atresia
   h. Megacolon
   i. Pelvic bone abnormalities
   j. IQ of 30 to 80

C. Interventions
1. Patient teaching (see *Patient with Down syndrome*)
2. Provide family with information regarding local, regional, and national organizations offering support to families and patients

◆ V. Phenylketonuria (PKU)

A. Pathophysiology
1. Inborn error in metabolism of the amino acid phenylalanine
2. Transmitted through an autosomal recessive gene
3. Patients with PKU have almost no hepatic phenylalanine hydroxylase, an enzyme that helps convert phenylalanine to tyrosine; therefore phenylalanine accumulates in blood and urine while tyrosine declines

4. Tyrosine is nonessential amino acid, a precursor for epinephrine, thyroxine, and melanin
5. If untreated, brain development is retarded and may be irreversible
6. To prevent this disorder, infants should be routinely screened for PKU

B. Assessment
1. Evidence of mental retardation by age 4 months
2. Personality disturbances
3. Seizures
4. Macrocephaly
5. Eczematous skin lesions or rough, dry skin
6. Hyperactivity, irritability
7. Repetitive movements
8. Musty odor from skin and urine

C. Interventions
1. Promote a diet restricted in protein to prevent excess accumulation of phenylalanine
2. Teach the parents to read food labels and to be especially aware of sweeteners, such as aspartame, which can contain phenylalanine

♦ VI. Sickle cell anemia

A. Pathophysiology
1. A congenital (autosomal recessive) hemolytic anemia that results from a defective hemoglobin molecule (hemoglobin S), which causes red blood cells (RBCs) to roughen and become sickle shaped
2. Damaged RBCs accumulate in capillaries and smaller blood vessels, increasing blood viscosity and causing occlusion
3. Impaired circulation results in chronic ill health, periodic acute crises, long-term complications, and premature death
4. Sickle cell (vaso-occlusive) crisis is triggered by conditions that cause cellular hypoxia: infection, cold exposure, high altitudes, overexertion
5. In crisis the sickle cells adhere to cell walls and to each other, blocking blood flow and causing areas of ischemia in organs and tissues, especially kidney and spleen, leading to tissue death
6. Affected individual may carry one gene for sickle cell anemia (sickle cell trait) or both genes (sickle cell disease)

B. Assessment
1. Signs and symptoms usually don't develop in infants until after age 6 months, because large amounts of fetal hemoglobin protect them
2. Chronic fatigue, unexplained dyspnea, dyspnea on exertion, joint swelling, aching bones, severe localized and generalized pain, leg ulcers, and frequent infections

3. In sickle cell crisis, signs and symptoms include severe pain, hematuria, lethargy, irritability, and pale lips, tongue, palms, and nail beds

C. Interventions
1. Sickle cell crisis
   a. Apply warm compresses to painful areas
   b. Administer an analgesic-antipyretic
   c. Encourage bed rest in a sitting position
   d. Administer antibiotics, as ordered
   e. Force fluids
2. During remission
   a. Advise patient to avoid tight clothing
   b. Warn against strenuous exercise
   c. Emphasize the need for prompt treatment of infection
   d. Advise the patient to increase fluid intake to prevent dehydration
3. During pregnancy or surgery
   a. Warn women that they may have increased obstetric risks
   b. During general anesthesia, patient requires optimal ventilation to prevent hypoxic crisis

◆ VII. Tay-Sach's disease

A. Pathophysiology
1. A congenital enzyme deficiency that causes progressive mental and motor deterioration and is always fatal, usually before age 5; prevalent among Ashkenazi (European) Jews
2. Autosomal recessive disorder in which the enzyme hexosaminidase A is deficient
3. Without hexosaminidase A, accumulating lipid pigments distend and progressively DEMYELINATE and destroy central nervous system cells

B. Assessment
1. Progressive weakness and flaccidity of the neck, trunk, arm, and leg muscles prevent infant from sitting up or lifting his head
2. Easily startled by sounds
3. By age 18 months, may have seizures, dementia, generalized paralysis, and spasticity
4. Vision loss progressing to blindness
5. By age 2, patient contracts bronchopneumonia, which is usually fatal
6. Enlarged head circumference
7. Distinctive cherry red spot on the retina

C. Interventions
   1. Supportive treatment such as tube feedings, postural drainage, and skin care
   2. Family education and support

POINTS TO REMEMBER

♦ Diagnosis of some genetic disorders can only be made through a thorough history and examination.

♦ Early diagnosis is essential in preventing irreversible damage in some disorders.

♦ Parent and patient education is an important part of nursing care in dealing with genetic disorders.

STUDY QUESTIONS

To evaluate your understanding of this chapter, answer the following questions in the space provided; then compare your responses with the correct answers in appendix B, page 294.

1. What is the best position for feeding an infant with cleft lip or cleft palate? _____

_____

2. Which enzymes are important for the patient with cystic fibrosis to take with meals? _____

_____

3. How many chromosomes does a patient with Down syndrome exhibit?

_____

_____

4. If not diagnosed and treated early, PKU can cause what condition to develop? _____

_____

5. Why doesn't sickle cell crisis begin to show signs and symptoms in a patient until age 6 months?_____

_____

6. What causes sickle cell crisis?_____

_____

CRITICAL THINKING AND APPLICATION EXERCISES

1. Prepare a patient education sheet on feeding for parents of an infant with cleft lip and/or cleft palate.

2. Develop a table showing autosomal dominant and autosomal recessive genes inheritance patterns.

3. Develop a diet plan for the patient with PKU.

4. Interview several patients with sickle cell anemia about how it affects their lives. Present your information to your fellow classmates for discussion about how to address the patient's issues.

5. Follow a patient with a genetic disorder from admission through discharge. Develop a patient-specific plan of care, including any needs for follow-up and rehabilitation.

Neoplasms

CHAPTER OVERVIEW

Knowledge of the ways in which normal cell growth can go awry provides the foundation for understanding how cancer begins, develops, and spreads throughout the body. Careful assessment and diagnostic tests are required to locate and correctly categorize the cancer. Nursing interventions aim to support the patient and maintain the patient's quality of life.

264

♦ I. Pathophysiologic processes

A. Cancer cells grow without the internal controls that characterize normal cells; may spread from site of origin in three ways
  1. By circulation through the blood and lymphatic system to distant tissue (metastasis)
  2. By accidental transplantation during surgery
  3. By invasion to adjacent organs and tissues

B. Carcinogenesis: cells change from normal to cancerous
  1. Probably results from a complex interaction between genetic factors and an initiator and a promoter substance that may include environmental agents
      a. Substances in the environment (carcinogens) can cause cancer by damaging cellular deoxyribonucleic acid
      b. Viruses can transform cells
      c. Overexposure to ultraviolet light or radiation may induce tumor development
      d. Diet and food additives
      e. Hormones: excessive use, especially estrogen, may contribute to some cancers while reducing the risks of others
  2. Immunologic incompetence
      a. Intact human immune system is responsible for spontaneous regression of tumors
      b. Inability of the body to recognize cancer cells as foreign allows the tumor to proliferate

♦ II. Malignant brain tumors

A. Pathophysiology
  1. Brain tumors cause central nervous system changes by invading and destroying tissues and by secondary effect
      a. Compression of the brain, cranial nerves and cerebral vessels
      b. Cerebral edema
      c. Increased intracranial pressure (ICP) (see *Comparing malignant brain tumors*, pages 266 to 268)
  2. Rarely metastasize to other parts of the body

B. Assessment
  1. Dependent on location, size, and rate of growth
  2. Signs and symptoms of ICP include headache, vomiting, pupillary dysfunction, motor dysfunction, papilledema, visual changes
  3. Seizures
  4. Personality changes
  5. Neurologic deficits specific to tumor location
  6. Cranial nerve dysfunction

(Text continues on page 268.)

Comparing malignant brain tumors

TUMOR	CLINICAL FEATURES
Astrocytoma • Second most common malignant glioma (approximately 80% of all gliomas) • Occurs at any age; incidence higher in males • Usually occurs in white matter of cerebral hemispheres; may originate in any part of the central nervous system • Cerebellar astrocytomas usually confined to one hemisphere	*General:* • Headache; mental activity changes • Decreased motor strength and coordination • Seizures; scanning speech • Altered vital signs *Localized:* • Third ventricle: changes in mental activity and level of consciousness, nausea, pupillary dilation and sluggish light reflex; later, paresis or ataxia • Brain stem and pons: early, ipsilateral trigeminal, abducens, and facial nerve palsies; later, cerebellar ataxia, tremors, other cranial nerve deficits • Third or fourth ventricle or aqueduct of Sylvius: secondary hydrocephalus • Thalamus or hydrothalamus: various endocrine, metabolic, autonomic, and behavioral changes
Glioblastoma multiforme (spongioblastoma multiforme; a type of astrocytoma) • Peak incidence between ages 50 and 60; twice as common in males; most common glioma • Unencapsulated; highly malignant; grows rapidly and infiltrates the brain extensively; may become enormous before diagnosed • Usually occurs in cerebral hemispheres, especially frontal and temporal lobes (rarely in brain stem and cerebellum) • Occupies more than one lobe of affected hemisphere; may spread to opposite hemisphere by corpus callosum; may metastasize into cerebrospinal fluid (CSF), producing tumors in distant parts of the nervous system	*General:* • Increased intracranial pressure (ICP), nausea, vomiting, headache, papilledema • Mental and behavioral changes • Altered vital signs (increased systolic pressure, widened pulse pressure, respiratory changes) • Speech and sensory disturbances • In children, irritability, projectile vomiting *Localized:* • Midline: headache (bifrontal or bioccipital); worse in the morning; intensified by coughing, straining, or sudden head movements • Temporal lobe: psychomotor seizures • Central region: focal seizures • Optic and oculomotor nerves: visual defects • Frontal lobes: abnormal reflexes, motor responses
Ependymoma • Rare glioma • Most common in children and young adults • Usually locates in fourth and lateral ventricles	*General:* • Similar to oligodendroglioma • Increased ICP and obstructive hydrocephalus, depending on tumor size

Comparing malignant brain tumors (continued)

TUMOR	CLINICAL FEATURES
Medulloblastoma • Rare glioma • Incidence highest in children ages 4 to 6 • Affects males more than females • Commonly metastasizes via CSF	*General:* • Increased ICP *Localized:* • Brain stem and cerebrum: papilledema, nystagmus, hearing loss, flashing lights, dizziness, ataxia, paresthesia of face, cranial nerve palsies (V, VI, VII,IX, X, primarily sensory), hemiparesis, suboccipital tenderness, compression of supratentorial area produces other general and focal signs and symptoms
Meningioma • Most common nongliomatous brain tumor (20% of primary brain tumors) • Peak incidence among 50-year-olds; rare in children; more common in females (ratio 3:2) • Arises from the meninges • Common locations include parasagittal area, sphenoid ridge, anterior part of the base of the skull, cerebellopontine angle, spinal canal • Benign, well-circumscribed, highly vascular tumors that compress underlying tissue by invading overlying skull	*General:* • Headache • Seizures (in two-thirds of patients) • Vomiting • Changes in mental activity • Similar to schwannomas *Localized:* • Skull changes (bony bulge) over tumor • Sphenoid ridge, indenting optic nerve: unilateral visual changes and papilledema • Prefrontal parasagittal area: personality and behavioral changes • Motor cortex: contralateral motor changes • Anterior fossa compressing both optic nerves and frontal lobes: headaches and bilateral vision loss • Pressure on cranial nerves causes varying symptoms
Oligodendroglioma • Third most common glioma (5%) • Occurs in middle adult years; more common in women • Slow-growing • Most common in cerebral hemispheres	*General:* • Mental and behavioral changes • Visual disturbances • Increased ICP *Localized:* • Temporal lobe: hallucinations, psychomotor seizures • Central region: seizures (confined to one muscle group or unilateral) • Midbrain or third ventricle: pyramidal tract symptoms (dizziness, ataxia, paresthesia of the face) • Brain stem and cerebrum: nystagmus, hearing loss, dizziness, ataxia, paresthesia of face, cranial nerve palsies, hemiparesis, suboccipital tenderness, loss of balance

(continued)

Comparing malignant brain tumors (continued)

TUMOR	CLINICAL FEATURES
Schwannoma (acoustic neurinoma, neurilemoma, cerebellopontine angle tumor) • Accounts for approximately 10% of all intracranial tumors • Higher incidence in women • Onset of symptoms between ages 30 and 60 • Affects the craniospinal nerve sheath, usually cranial nerve VIII; also, V and VII; and to a lesser extent, VI and X on the same side as the tumor • Benign, but commonly classified as malignant because of its growth patterns; slow-growing; may be present for years before symptoms occur	*General:* • Unilateral hearing loss with or without tinnitus • Stiff neck and suboccipital discomfort • Secondary hydrocephalus • Ataxia and uncoordinated movements of one or both arms due to pressure on brain stem and cerebellum *Localized:* • V: early-facial hypoesthesia/paresthesia on side of hearing loss; unilateral loss of corneal reflex • VI: diplopia or double vision • VII: paresis progressing to paralysis (Bell's palsy) • X: weakness of palate, tongue, and nerve muscles on same side as tumor

C. Interventions
1. Removing a resectable tumor; radiation therapy
2. Reducing a nonresectable tumor; radiation therapy; chemotherapy
3. Relieving cerebral edema, increased ICP
4. Preventing further neurologic damage
5. Postoperative care
   a. Maintain patent airway
   b. Maintain patient safety
   c. Administer anticonvulsant drugs, as prescribed

CLINICAL ALERT

   d. Check continuously for changes in neurologic status, and watch for increased ICP
   e. Maintain normal fluid volume and electrolyte imbalance
6. Teach the patient and his family symptoms of recurrence; urge compliance with treatment regimen
7. Brain tumors may cause residual neurologic deficits that disable the patient; begin rehabilitation early

◆ III. Lung cancer

A. Pathophysiology
1. Four common types
   a. Adenocarcinoma
   b. Squamous (epidermoid)

    c. Large cell (anaplastic)

    d. Small cell (oat cell)

2. Lung cancer most commonly results from inhalation of irritants or carcinogens (such as coal dust, tobacco, asbestos)

3. In normal lungs, the epithelium lines and protects the tissue below it; when exposed to irritants or carcinogens, epithelium becomes DYSPLASTIC

4. Dysplastic cells lose protective function, exposing underlying cells to carcinogens

5. Eventually, the dysplastic cells turn into neoplastic carcinoma and start invading deeper tissues (see *Common lung cancers,* page 270)

6. Sites of metastases include brain, bone, liver

B. Assessment

1. Smoker's cough (chronic)

2. Hoarseness, dysphagia

3. Wheezing

4. Dyspnea

5. Hemoptysis

6. Chest and shoulder pain

7. Fever

8. Weakness

9. Weight loss

10. Anorexia

11. Superior vena cava syndrome

12. Pleural effusion

C. Interventions

1. Surgery (lobectomy, pneumonectomy, segmental resection)

    a. Postoperative care

      (1) Maintain a patent airway and monitor chest tubes

      (2) Monitor vital signs and fluid intake and output

      (3) Watch for and treat infection, shock, hemorrhage, atelectasis, dyspnea, mediastinal shift, and pulmonary embolus

      (4) To prevent pulmonary embolus, apply antiembolism stockings and encourage range-of-motion exercises

2. Radiation and chemotherapy

    a. Explain possible adverse effects; watch for these effects and treat them

    b. Diet: soft, nonirritating foods that are high in protein and high-calorie between-meal snacks

    c. Administer antiemetics and antidiarrheals, as needed

    d. Provide good skin care

Common lung cancers

The table below describes the growth rate, metastasis sites, diagnostic tests, signs and symptoms, for four common lung cancers.

TYPE OF CANCER	RATE OF GROWTH	METASTASIS	SIGNS AND SYMPTOMS	DIAGNOSTIC TESTS
Adenocarcinoma	• Moderate	• Early metastasis	• Pleural effusion	• Fiberoptic bronchoscopy, radiography, electron microscopy
Squamous (epidermoid)	• Slow	• Late metastasis mainly to hilar lymph nodes, chest wall, and mediastinum	• Airway obstruction, cough, sputum production	• Sputum analysis, biopsy, immunohistochemistry, electron microscopy, bronchoscopy
Large cell (anaplastic)	• Fast	• Early, extensive metastasis	• Cough, hemoptysis, chest wall pain, pleural effusion, sputum production, pneumonia-induced airway obstruction	• Bronchoscopy, sputum analysis, electron microscopy
Small cell (oat cell)	• Very fast	• Very early metastasis to mediastinum, hilar lymph nodes, and other organ sites	• Chest pain, cough, hemoptysis, dyspnea, localized wheezing, pneumonia-induced airway obstruction, muscle weakness, facial edema, hypokalemia, hyperglycemia, hypertension, and other signs and symptoms related to excessive hormone secretion	• Sputum analysis, immunohistochemistry, electron microscopy, bronchoscopy

◆ IV. Breast cancer

A. Pathophysiology

1. Adenocarcinoma: most common form, arises from the epithelial tissues

TEACHING TIPS
Patient with breast cancer

Be sure to include the following topics in your teaching plan for the patient with breast cancer:
• Instruct the patient about breast prostheses.
• Provide emotional and psychological support.
• Inform the patient about support groups.
• Urge the patient to have a mammogram at least once a year, and to conduct a self-breast exam each month.
• If appropriate, teach the patient postmastectomy exercises to prevent lymph-edema

2. Intraductal: develops within the ducts
3. Infiltrating: arises in the parenchyma
4. Inflammatory: cancer grows rapidly and causes the overlying skin to become edematous, inflamed, and indurated
5. Lobular: involves the lobes of glandular tissue
6. Medullary or circumscribed: a tumor that grows rapidly

B. Assessment
1. Palpable, painless lump or mass
2. Change in symmetry or size of the breast
3. Nipple retraction; scaly skin around the nipple; clear, milky, or bloody discharge
4. Change in skin temperature (warm, hot or pink area); skin puckering
5. Edema of the arm

C. Interventions
1. Surgery: lumpectomy, mastectomy, node dissection
2. Postoperative care
   a. Inspect dressings, report bleeding promptly
   b. Measure and record the amount of drainage
   c. Check circulatory status
   d. Monitor fluids
   e. Prevent lymphedema of the arm by exercising and avoiding activities that might cause infection
   f. Advise the patient to discuss reconstructive surgery with her doctor
3. Patient education (see *Patient with breast cancer*)
4. Peripheral stem cell therapy
5. Primary radiation therapy before or after tumor removal

      6. Hormonal manipulation (for example, estrogen, progesterone, an-
         drogen, or antiandrogen therapy)
      7. Genetic counseling

◆ V. Pancreatic cancer

  A. Pathophysiology
      1. A deadly cancer, pancreatic cancer progresses rapidly
      2. Most pancreatic tumors are adenocarcinomas and arise in the head
         of the pancreas
      3. Rarer tumors are those of the body and tail of the pancreas and islet
         cell tumors (see *Comparing types of pancreatic cancer*)
      4. Possible predisposing factors include smoking, chronic pancreatitis,
         diabetes mellitus, chronic alcohol abuse, and diet high in fat or meat
         or both

  B. Assessment
      1. Weight loss
      2. Abdominal or low back pain
      3. Jaundice
      4. Diarrhea
      5. Pruritus

  C. Interventions
      1. Treatment is rarely successful because this disease has usually metas-
         tasized widely by the time it has been diagnosed
      2. Surgery
        a. Total pancreatectomy
        b. Cholecystojejunostomy, choledochoduodenectomy, and choledo-
          chojejunostomy
        c. Whipple's operation or pancreatoduodenectomy
        d. Gastrojejunostomy
      3. Chemotherapy
      4. Radiation therapy
      5. Administer prescribed medications
        a. Antibiotics
        b. Anticholinergics
        c. Antacids
        d. Diuretics
        e. Insulin
        f. Narcotics
        g. Pancreatic enzymes

◆ VI. Colorectal cancer

  A. Pathophysiology
      1. Colorectal malignant tumors are almost always adenocarcinomas
      2. About half of these are SESSILE lesions; the rest are polypoid

Comparing types of pancreatic cancer

TYPE AND PATHOLOGY	CLINICAL FEATURES
Head of pancreas • Commonly obstructs ampulla of Vater and common bile duct • Directly metastasizes to duodenum • Adhesions anchor tumor to spine, stomach, and intestines	• Jaundice (predominant sign) — slowly progressive, unremitting; may cause skin (especially of the face and genitals) to turn olive green or black • Pruritus — in many cases severe • Weight loss — rapid and severe (as great as 30 lb [13.5 kg]); may lead to emaciation, weakness, and muscle atrophy • Slowed digestion, gastric distention, nausea, diarrhea, and steatorrhea with clay-colored stools • Liver and gallbladder enlargement from lymph node metastasis to biliary tract and duct wall results in compression and obstruction; gallbladder may be palpable (Courvoisier's sign) • Dull, nondescript, continuous abdominal pain radiating to right upper quadrant; relieved by bending forward • GI hemorrhage and biliary infection common
Body and tail of pancreas • Large nodular masses become fixed to retropancreatic tissues and spine • Direct invasion of spleen, left kidney, suprarenal gland, diaphragm • Involvement of celiac plexus results in thrombosis of splenic vein and spleen infarction	*Body:* • Pain (predominant symptom) — usually epigastric, develops slowly and radiates to back; relieved by bending forward or sitting up; intensified by lying supine; most intense 3 to 4 hours after eating; when celiac plexus is involved, pain is more intense and lasts longer • Venous thrombosis and thrombophlebitis — common; may precede other symptoms by months • Splenomegaly (from infarction), hepatomegaly (occasionally), and jaundice (rarely) *Tail:* *Signs and symptoms result from metastasis:* • Abdominal tumor (most common finding) produces a palpable abdominal mass; abdominal pain radiates to left hypochondrium and left side of the chest • Anorexia leads to weight loss, emaciation, and weakness • Splenomegaly and upper GI bleeding

3. Tends to progress slowly and remain localized for a long time

4. High-fat, low-fiber diet may contribute to colorectal cancer by slowing fecal movement through the bowel

5. This results in prolonged exposure of the bowel mucosa to digested toxins and carcinogens and may encourage mucosal cells to mutate

B. Assessment

1. Right-side tumor
   a. Abdominal aching
   b. Cramps
   c. Black, tarry stool
   d. In many cases, palpation of the abdomen reveals a mass
2. Left-side tumor
   a. Change in bowel habit, such as diarrhea or constipation
   b. Rectal bleeding
   c. Bloody stools
   d. Nausea, vomiting
   e. Intermittent abdominal fullness, cramping and rectal pressure

C. Interventions

1. Surgery: depends on location of the tumor; may involve temporary or permanent ostomy
2. Chemotherapy: used for patients with metastasis, residual disease, or a recurrent inoperable tumor
3. Radiation therapy

◆ VII. Liver cancer

A. Pathophysiology

1. A rare form of primary cancer with a high mortality rate
2. Some primary tumors originate in the parenchymal cells and are hepatomas (related to chronic infection with the hepatitis B virus, cirrhosis, and hepatocarcinogens in food)
3. Other primary tumors originate in the intrahepatic bile ducts and are cholangiomas
4. The liver is one of the most common sites of metastasis from other primary cancers, particularly those of colon, rectum, stomach, esophagus, lung, breast, and skin

B. Assessment

1. A mass in the right upper quadrant; bloating or abdominal fullness
2. Tender, nodular liver on palpation
3. Dull, aching pain in the epigastrium or the right upper quadrant
4. Bruit, hum, or rubbing sound if tumor involves a large part of the liver
5. Weight loss, weakness, anorexia, fever
6. Occasional jaundice or ascites

7. Occasional evidence of metastasis through venous system to lungs, from lymphatics to regional lymph nodes, or by direct invasion of portal veins
8. Dependent edema

C. Interventions
1. Radiation therapy
2. Chemotherapy
3. Liver transplantation for some patients; subtotal hepatectomy
4. Control edema and ascites
5. Diet: restrict fat, sodium, fluids, and protein
6. Monitor respiratory function (bilateral pleural effusion is common)
7. Relieve fever with aspirin; avoid acetaminophen because the diseased liver can't metabolize it
8. Give meticulous skin care

♦ VIII. Prostatic cancer

A. Pathophysiology
1. Most common cancer in men over age 50; most prevalent among African-American men
2. Most prostatic carcinomas originate in the posterior prostate gland; the rest originate near the urethra
3. Malignant tumors seldom result from the benign prostatic hyperplasia that commonly develops around the urethra in elderly men (see chapter 13, for more on the disorder)
4. When primary lesions spread beyond the prostate gland, they invade the prostatic capsule and then spread along the ejaculatory ducts in the space between the seminal vesicles or perivesicular fascia

B. Assessment
1. Seldom produces symptoms until well advanced
2. Slow urine stream
3. Urinary hesitancy
4. Incomplete bladder emptying
5. Dysuria; nocturia, urgency
6. Hematuria

C. Interventions
1. Surgery: radical prostatectomy, orchiectomy
2. Radiation therapy (watch for common adverse effects: prostatitis, diarrhea, bladder spasms, and urinary frequency)
3. Androgen-deprivation therapy (orchiectomy, luteinizing hormone–releasing hormone analogues, antiandrogens, adrenal androgen inhibitors)
4. Chemotherapy

◆ IX. Cervical cancer

A. Pathophysiology
1. Classified as either preinvasive or invasive
   a. Preinvasive: ranges from minimal cervical dysplasia to carcinoma in situ, in which the full thickness of epithelium contains abnormal cells
   b. Invasive: cancer cells penetrate the basement membrane and can spread directly to pelvic structures or disseminate by lymphatic routes
2. Considered a sexually transmitted disease associated with human papillomavirus

B. Assessment
1. May produce no early symptoms
2. Abnormal vaginal bleeding
3. Persistent vaginal discharge
4. Postcoital pain and bleeding

C. Interventions
1. Excisional biopsy: patient may feel pressure, minor abdominal cramps, or a pinch from punch forceps
2. Cryosurgery: procedure takes 15 minutes; doctor uses refrigerant to freeze the cervix; patient may experience abdominal cramps, headache and sweating, but little if any pain
3. Laser therapy: may cause abdominal cramping
4. Therapeutic conization
5. Hysterectomy (extended or radical); pelvic node dissection; pelvic exenteration
6. Radiation therapy: internal or external therapy
   a. Internal (intracavity)
      (1) Enforce radiation safety precautions
      (2) Encourage patient to limit movement while the source is in place
   b. External: continues for 4 to 6 weeks as outpatient
7. Teach patient to watch for adverse effects such as infections
8. Teach patient how to use a vaginal dilator to prevent vaginal stenosis

◆ X. Uterine (endometrial) cancer

A. Pathophysiology
1. Cancer of the endometrium is the most common gynecologic cancer
2. In most cases, it is an adenocarcinoma that metastasizes late, usually from the endometrium to the cervix, ovaries, fallopian tubes, and other peritoneal structures

3. Predisposing factors
   a. Prolonged estrogen exposure (early menarche, late menopause, no pregnancy, anovulation)
   b. Obesity, hypertension, diabetes, or polycystic ovaries
   c. Familial tendency
   d. History of uterine polyps or endometrial hyperplasia
   e. Estrogen therapy (still controversial)
   f. Estrogen-secreting ovarian tumors

B. Assessment
1. Uterine enlargement
2. Persistent and unusual premenopausal bleeding
3. Any postmenopausal bleeding

C. Interventions
1. Surgery: total abdominal hysterectomy with bilateral oophorectomy and sampling regional lymph nodes
2. Radiation therapy: external or internal
   a. Internal
     (1) Enforce radiation safety precautions
     (2) Encourage patient to limit movement while the source is in place
   b. External
     (1) Teach the patient how to use a vaginal dilator to prevent vaginal stenosis
     (2) Treatments last 4 to 6 weeks
     (3) Watch for infections

◆ XI. Ovarian cancer

A. Pathophysiology
1. Second most common female genitourinary cancer, and most lethal
2. Three main types
   a. Primary epithelial tumors arise in the epithelium
   b. Germ cell tumors in the ovum itself
   c. Sex cord–stromal tumors in the ovarian stroma
3. Ovarian tumors spread rapidly intraperitoneally by local extension or surface seeding and, occasionally, through the lymphatics and the bloodstream

B. Assessment
1. Vague abdominal discomfort, bloating, flatulence, dyspepsia, and other mild GI disturbances
2. Urinary frequency, constipation, pelvic discomfort, distention, and weight loss
3. Postmenopausal bleeding and pain
4. Ascites

C. Interventions
   1. Surgery: total abdominal hysterectomy with bilateral salpingo oophorectomy; removal of omentum, sampling liver, diaphragm, retroperitoneal, and aortic lymph nodes as well as peritoneal surface
   2. Chemotherapy; extends survival time and is largely palliative

♦ XII. Leukemia

A. Pathophysiology
   1. A group of malignant blood disorders marked by abnormal proliferation and maturation of lymphocytes and non-lymphocytic cells in the bone marrow, leading to suppression of normal cells (erythrocytes, thrombocytes, uninvolved white blood cells [WBCs])
   2. Two classifications
      a. Chronic or acute
      b. Myeloid or lymphoid
   3. Risk factors for developing leukemia
      a. Chromosomal abnormalities (such as Down syndrome, trisomy-13, Philadelphia chromosome)
      b. Exposure to large doses of ionizing radiation or drugs that suppress the bone marrow
      c. Exposure to viruses, such as human T-cell lymphotropic virus type 1

B. Assessment
   1. Symptoms of acute lymphocytic leukemia (ALL) and acute myelogenous leukemia (AML) are similar
      a. Repeated infection
      b. Bleeding
      c. Anemia
      d. Malaise, fever, lethargy
      e. Weight loss
      f. Night sweats
      g. Generalized lymphadenopathy
      h. Splenomegaly, hepatomegaly
      i. Bone, joint pain
      j. Central nervous system: headache, nausea and vomiting, cranial nerve palsies, papilledema, coma, seizures
   2. Symptoms of chronic myelogenous leukemia (CML)
      a. Fatigue, weakness
      b. Weight loss
      c. Heat intolerance
      d. Increased diaphoresis
      e. Splenomegaly with abdominal fullness
      f. Bleeding and bruising due to low platelet count
      g. Exertional dyspnea

h. Onset of "blast crisis": revert to AML
3. Symptoms of chronic lymphocytic leukemia (CLL)
   a. Fever
   b. Frequent infections
   c. Fatigue
   d. Enlargement of lymph nodes
   e. Splenomegaly

C. Interventions
   1. Three-stage treatment of ALL
      a. Induction therapy: vincristine, prednisone, and L-asparaginase, plus an anthracycline for adults
      b. CNS prophylaxis: intrathecal methotrexate and intracranial radiation
      c. Postremission therapy: high-dose chemotherapy (intensification) followed by 2 to 3 years of maintenance chemotherapy
   2. Two-stage treatment of AML
      a. Induction therapy: cytarabine and an anthracycline
      b. Postremission therapy: intensification, maintenance chemotherapy, or bone marrow transplantation
   3. Treatment of CML
      a. Goal is to control leukocytosis and thrombocytosis
      b. Busulfan and hydroxyurea
      c. Bone marrow transplantation
      d. Local splenic radiation or splenectomy
      e. Leukapheresis
      f. Interferon therapy
      g. Aspirin to prevent cerebrovascular accident
      h. Allopurinol and colchicine to prevent or relieve gout
   4. Treatment of CLL
      a. For autoimmune hemolytic anemia or thrombocytopenia: systemic chemotherapy (chlorambucil or cyclophosphamide) or prednisone
      b. For organ obstruction, impairment, or enlargement: local radiation, splenectomy
      c. Radiation therapy for enlarged lymph nodes, painful bony lesions, massive splenomegaly
      d. Allopurinol to prevent hyperuricemia

◆ XIII. Primary malignant bone cancer

A. Pathophysiology
   1. Also called sarcomas of the bone and bone cancer
   2. May originate in the osseous or nonosseous tissues
      a. Osseous tumors arise from the bony structure itself
      b. Nonosseous tumors arise from hematopoetic, vascular and neural tissues (see *Comparing primary malignant bone tumors*, pages 280 and 281)

Comparing primary malignant bone tumors

TYPE	CLINICAL FEATURES	TREATMENT
Osseous origin Chondrosarcoma	• Develops from cartilage • Painless; grows slowly but is locally recurrent and invasive • Occurs most commonly in pelvis, proximal femur, ribs, and shoulder girdle • Usually in males between ages 30 and 50	• Hemipelvectomy, surgical resection (ribs) • Radiation (palliative) • Chemotherapy
Malignant giant cell tumor	• Arises from benign giant cell tumor • Found most commonly in long bones, especially in knee area • Usually in females between ages 18 and 50	• Curettage • Total excision • Radiation for recurrent disease
Osteogenic sarcoma	• Osteoid tumor present in specimen • Tumor arises from bone-forming osteoblasts and bone-digesting osteoclasts • Occurs most commonly in femur but also in tibia and humerus; occasionally in fibula, ileum, vertebra, or mandible • Usually in males between ages 10 and 30	• Surgery (tumor resection, high thigh amputation, hemipelvectomy, interscapulothoracic surgery) • Chemotherapy
Parosteal osteogenic sarcoma	• Develops on surface of bone instead of interior • Progresses slowly • Occurs most commonly in distal femur but also in tibia, humerus, and ulna • Usually in females between ages 30 and 40	• Surgery (tumor resection, possible amputation, interscapulothoracic surgery, hemipelvectomy) • Chemotherapy • Combination of above
Nonosseous origin Chordoma	• Derived from embryonic remnants of notochord • Progresses slowly	• Surgical resection (may result in neural defects) • Radiation (palliative, or when surgery not applicable, as in occipital area)

Comparing primary malignant bone tumors (continued)

TYPE	CLINICAL FEATURES	TREATMENT
Nonosseous origin Chordoma *(continued)*	• Usually found at end of spinal column and in spheno-occipital, sacro-coccygeal, and vertebral areas • Characterized by constipation and visual disturbances • Usually in males between ages 50 and 60	• Radiation (palliative, or when surgery not applicable, as in occipital area)
Ewing's sarcoma	• Originates in bone marrow and invades shafts of long and flat bones • Usually affects lower extremities, most commonly femur, innominate bones, ribs, tibia, humerus, vertebra, and fibula; may metastasize to lungs • Pain increasingly severe and persistent • Usually in males between ages 10 and 20 • Prognosis poor	• High-voltage radiation (tumor is radiosensitive) • Chemotherapy to slow growth • Amputation only if there's no evidence of metastases
Fibrosarcoma	• Relatively rare • Originates in fibrous tissue of bone • Invades long or flat bones (femur, tibia, mandible) but also involves periosteum and overlying muscle • Usually in males between ages 30 and 40	• Amputation • Radiation • Chemotherapy • Bone grafts (with low-grade fibrosarcoma)

B. Assessment
1. Bone pain, more intense at night and not associated with mobility
2. Presence of a mass or tumor
3. Pathologic fractures
4. Limitation of movement
5. Decreased sensation

C. Interventions

1. Wide excision of the tumor or amputation
2. Intensive chemotherapy
3. Radiation therapy
4. Provide emotional support for the strain caused by threat of amputation

♦XIV. Basal cell carcinoma

A. Pathophysiology

1. A slow-growing, destructive skin tumor
2. Most common skin cancer
3. Usually occurs in blond, fair-skinned males over age 40 with a history of significant long-term sun exposure
4. Three types
   a. Nodulo-ulcerative carcinomas occur on the face, particularly the forehead, eyelid margins, and nasolabial folds
   b. Superficial basal cell carcinomas are multiple and mostly occur on the chest and back
   c. Sclerosing basal cell carcinomas occur on the head and neck

B. Assessment

1. Nodulo-ulcerative lesions are small, smooth, pinkish, and translucent
2. Superficial basal cell lesions are oval, irregularly shaped, lightly pigmented plaques, with sharply defined, elevated threadlike borders
3. Sclerosing basal cell lesions are waxy, sclerotic, yellow to white plaques without distinct borders

C. Interventions

1. Curettage and electrodissection
2. Topical 5-fluorouracil (chemosurgery)
3. Surgical excision
4. Irradiation
5. Cryotherapy
6. Teach patient to prevent recurrence by avoiding sun exposure and using a strong sunscreen

♦XV. Malignant melanoma

A. Pathophysiology

1. Arises from melanocytes (cells that synthesize the pigment melanin)
2. Besides the skin, melanocytes are found in the meninges, alimentary canal, respiratory tract, lymph nodes
3. Melanoma spreads through the lymphatic and vascular systems and metastasizes to the regional lymph nodes, skin, liver, lungs, and CNS

B. Assessment
  1. Look for any preexisting lesion or nevus that enlarges, changes color or texture, becomes inflamed or sore, itches, ulcerates, bleeds, or shows sign of surrounding pigment regression
  2. Use the ABCD rule: Look for <u>A</u>symmetry, an irregular <u>B</u>order, <u>C</u>olor variation, and a <u>D</u>iameter greater than ¼″ (6 mm)
C. Interventions
  1. Screening; regular self-examination
  2. Wide surgical resection with skin graft to remove the tumor
  3. Chemotherapy, radiation therapy, immunotherapy
  4. Emphasize the need for close follow-ups to detect recurrences early
  5. Urge meticulous use of sun-blocking agents

◆ XVI. Kaposi's sarcoma

A. Pathophysiology
  1. Cancer of the endothelial cells that line small blood vessels
  2. Most common acquired immunodeficiency syndrome–related cancer; tumor nodules appear first on head, neck, and trunk; progresses aggressively, involving the lymph nodes, lungs, and GI structures
B. Assessment
  1. One or more obvious lesions in various shapes, sizes, and colors (ranging from red-brown to dark purple)
  2. Appears most commonly on the skin, buccal mucosa, hard and soft palate, lips, gums, tongue, tonsils, conjunctiva, and sclera
C. Interventions
  1. Radiation therapy
  2. Chemotherapy
  3. Follow standard precautions
  4. Provide emotional support
  5. Diet: high-calorie, high-protein
  6. Administer pain medications, as ordered
  7. Monitor patient's weight daily
  8. Refer patient to support groups

POINTS TO REMEMBER

◆ Early detection of cancer enables more effective treatment and a better prognosis.

◆ When gathering assessment information, ask the patient about risk factors, family history, and exposure to potential hazards.

STUDY QUESTIONS

To evaluate your understanding of this chapter, answer the following questions in the space provided; then compare your responses with the correct answers in appendix B, page 294.

1. What are some signs and symptoms of increased ICP? _____

    _____

2. What is the most common form of breast cancer?_____

    _____

3. What type of diet is thought to contribute to colorectal cancer? _____

    _____

4. What are some important teaching tips for patients to prevent skin cancers? _____

    _____

5. What may a change in the shape, color, and texture of a nevus indicate?

    _____

    _____

CRITICAL THINKING AND APPLICATION EXERCISES

1. Prepare a drug card for tamoxifen.

2. Attend a breast cancer support group. Discuss your observations with your classmates.

3. Develop a chart showing the risk factors for breast cancer.

4. Observe an amputee patient in physical therapy. Discuss what you observed with your classmates.

5. Follow a cancer patient from admission through discharge. Develop a patient-specific plan of care, including any needs for follow-up and patient teaching.

Glossary

Acid—substance with excess hydrogen ions and a pH under 7.0

Akinesia—absence of movements

Allergen—substance that induces an allergy or hypersensitivity reaction

Alveoli—hollow cellular lung structures that hold air

Anaphylaxis—severe allergic reaction to a foreign substance

Antibodies—proteins of high molecular weight (immunoglobulins) that are produced by B cells in response to specific antigens

Antigens—foreign substances, such as bacteria or toxins, that induce antibody formation

Apheresis—procedure in which blood is withdrawn from a donor, one or more components is removed, and the remainder is returned to the donor

Arthralgia—joint pain

Asynergia—lack of coordination of parts that normally act in harmony

Autoinoculation—inoculation with organisms from one's own body

Bone marrow—soft organic tissue found in the cavities of bones

Borborygmus—rumbling sound that occurs when gas is propelled through the intestines

Brudzinski's sign—assessment technique used to determine the presence of meningitis; it is considered positive when forward flexion of the neck causes hip and knee flexion

Bruit—sound of abnormal blood flow heard on auscultation

Bursa—fluid-filled sac found in connecting tissue in the vicinity of joints at likely friction points

Cardiac output—amount of blood ejected from the heart per minute

Cartilage—dense connective tissue consisting of fibers embedded in a strong gel-like substance; supports, cushions, and shapes body structures

Cells—smallest living components of an organism; the body's basic building blocks

Cerebrum—largest section of the brain, divided into two hemispheres by the longitudinal fissure; performs sensory, motor, and integrative functions related to mental activities

Chancre—small, dry or fluid-filled lesion; a primary sore or ulcer at the site of entry of an infectious organism

Cholestasis—interruption or decrease in bile flow

Cholesteatoma—cystlike mass most commonly occurring in the middle ear and mastoid

Clearance—complete removal of a substance by the kidneys from a specific volume of blood per unit of time

Common bile duct—duct that receives bile from the hepatic and cystic ducts and transports it to the duodenum

Crackles—abnormal inspiratory or expiratory breath sounds, usually associated with the presence of pleural fluid

Crepitation—dry, crackling sound or sensation that is present, for example, when ends of a broken bone are moved or when calculi are found in the prostate upon palpation

Cryptogenic—of questionable origin

Demyelinate—to remove the protective myelin sheath of a nerve cell

Deoxyribonucleic acid (DNA)—complex protein located in chromosomes in the cell's nucleus; carries genetic material and controls cellular reproduction

Digestion—breakdown of foods into absorbable nutrients in the gastrointestinal tract

Diverticulum—a blind pouch opening off another organ, such as the intestine

Dyskinesia—impairment of voluntary movement

Dysplastic—altered in size, shape, and organization; marked by abnormal growth or development

Dyspnea—difficult, labored breathing

Embolism—sudden obstruction of a blood vessel by foreign substances, a blood clot, or an air bubble

Exogenous—occurring outside the body

Glomerulus—a network of interconnected capillaries in the nephron, the basic unit of the kidney; brings blood and waste products carried by blood to the nephron

Hematemesis—vomiting of blood

Hemolysis—destruction of red blood cells

Homeostasis—dynamic, steady state of internal balance between different elements or groups of elements in the body

Hormone—chemical transmitter released from specialized cells into the bloodstream; produces a stimulatory effect on the targeted tissue

Host defense system—complex system consisting of antigens, antibodies, complement, and various types of white blood cells such as B and T lymphocytes. These elements interact to protect the host from pathogens.

Hyperemia—excess of blood in a body part; congestion

Hyperplasia—excessive growth of normal cells, causing an increase in the volume of a tissue or organ

Hyphema—blood in the front chamber of the eye

Immunoglobulin—serum protein synthesized by lymphocytes and plasma cells that has known antibody activity; main component of humoral immune response

Intermittent claudication—calf pain caused by walking and relieved by rest — for example, in Buerger's disease

Ischemia—decreased blood supply to a body organ or tissue

Joint—site of the union of two or more bones; provides motion and flexibility

Kernig's sign—assessment technique used to determine the presence of meningitis; considered positive when attempts to flex the hip of a patient in a recumbent position produce painful spasms of the hamstring mus-

cle and resistance to further leg extension at the knee

Lymphocyte—leukocyte produced by stem cells and matured in lymphoid tissue that participates in immune reactions

Macrophage—highly phagocytic cell that is stimulated by inflammation

Melena—black, tarry stools

Meninges—connective tissue membranes that enclose the brain and spinal cord; the three meninges are the dura mater, arachnoid, and pia mater

Micrographia—loss of fine motor control

Myalgia—muscle pain

Nephron—structural and functional unit of the kidney that forms urine

Odynophagia—pain caused by the act of swallowing

Opportunistic infection—infection that develops in people with altered, weakened immune systems; caused by a microorganism that doesn't ordinarily cause disease but becomes pathogenic under favorable conditions

Orthopnea—respiratory distress that is relieved by sitting upright

Osteoblasts—bone-forming cells

Osteoclasts—giant multinuclear cells that resorb material from previously formed bones, tear down old or excess bone structure, and allow osteoblasts to rebuild new bone

Papilloma—benign tumor that arises from skin, mucous membranes, or glandular ducts

Pathogen—disease-producing agent or microorganism

Phagocytosis—engulfing of foreign particles by cells called phagocytes

Photopsia—recurrent flashes of light caused by retinal irritation

Proteolytic enzymes—enzymes that promote splitting of proteins by hydrolysis of peptide bonds

Pyogenic—generating pus

Rhonchi—abnormal inspiratory or expiratory breath sounds, usually associated with airway constriction

Rigors—chills

Sessile—attached directly on a broad base; not stalked

Stasis—stoppage of the normal flow of fluids, such as blood and urine, or of digested matter within the intestinal system

Stenosis—constriction or narrowing of a passage or orifice

Synovial fluid—viscous, lubricating substance secreted by the synovial membrane, which lines the cavity between the bones of free-moving joints

Synovitis—inflammation of the synovial membrane

Tachypnea—abnormally fast rate of breathing

Tendon—fibrous cord of connective tissue that attaches the muscle to the bone or cartilage and enables bones to move when skeletal muscles contract

Tenesmus—painful straining at stool

Teratogen—substance capable of producing abnormalities during development

Tubercles—tiny nodules surrounded by lymphocytes; characteristic lesions of tuberculosis

Uremic frost—white, flaky deposits of urea on the skin of patients with advanced uremia

Virus—microscopic, infectious parasite that contains genetic material and needs a host to replicate

Answers to Study Questions

CHAPTER 1

1. The signs and symptoms of right- and left-sided heart failure include the following: fatigue, malaise, weakness, exertional and paroxysmal nocturnal dyspnea, tachypnea, neck vein engorgement, hepatojugular reflux, marked hepatomegaly, splenomegaly, tachycardia, palpitations, dependent pitting edema, unexplained steady weight gain, nausea, anorexia, abdominal fullness, ascites, chest tightness, slowed mental response, restlessness, hypotension, narrow pulse pressure, gallop rhythms S_3 and S_4 (third and fourth heart sounds), inspiratory crackles on auscultation, cough, cyanosis, and diaphoresis.

2. Four causes of hypovolemic shock include GI bleeding, internal hemorrhage (such as hemothorax), external hemorrhage (such as accident-related or surgical trauma), and any condition that reduces the volume of circulating intravascular plasma or other body fluids (such as severe burns, diarrhea, vomiting, dehydration, or third spacing).

3. Beck's triad consists of three signs characteristic of cardiac tamponade: elevated central venous pressure with neck vein distention, muffled heart sounds, and paradoxical pulse (inspiratory drop in systolic blood pressure greater than 15 mm Hg).

4. Cardiac tamponade's major pathophysiologic effect is distention of the pericardium as it fills with fluid.

5. Assessment findings in acute pulmonary edema include dyspnea; paroxysmal cough; blood-tinged, frothy sputum; orthopnea; tachycardia; agitation; restlessness; chest pain; syncope; tachycardia; cold, clammy skin; and gallop rhythms S_3 and S_4 (third and fourth heart sounds).

CHAPTER 2

1. Aneurysms are classified as saccular, fusiform, dissecting, or false.

2. Aneurysms most commonly occur in the ascending aorta, located in the thorax.

3. Three predisposing factors for deep vein thrombosis are prolonged bed rest, trauma, surgery, and childbirth.

CHAPTER 3

1. Cardiac-related causes of pulmonary edema include atherosclerosis, myocardial infarction, heart failure, overload of I.V. flu-

ids, or vasculitis. Noncardiac causes include ARDS, severe neurologic injury, and high altitudes.

2. Pneumothorax is classified as spontaneous, traumatic, or tension.
3. Assessment findings in pneumonia include cough, shortness of breath, chills, dyspnea, elevated temperature, crackles, rhonchi, pleural friction rub, pleuritic pain, and sputum production.
4. Chronic bronchitis is caused by inhaling airborne pollutants (especially by smoking) over a prolonged period, which stimulates excessive bronchial mucus production.

CHAPTER 4

1. Platelets minimize blood loss by providing materials that interact with plasma to accelerate blood coagulation.
2. Thrombocytopenia may be treated by treating the underlying cause; administering corticosteroids, folate, gamma globulin, or platelets; or performing splenectomy.
3. Disseminated intravascular coagulation is the body's response to an injury or disease in which microthrombi obstruct the blood supply to organs and hemorrhage occurs throughout the body. Activation of the thrombin and fibrinolytic system results in simultaneous bleeding and thrombosis.
4. In idiopathic thrombocytopenic purpura, antibody-coated platelets are phagocytized and removed from the circulation by

the reticuloendothelial cells of the spleen and liver. This cumulative loss of circulating platelets causes bleeding.

CHAPTER 5

1. The two compensatory mechanisms that protect the brain under adverse conditions are collateral circulation, which seeks to maintain adequate blood flow if normal blood flow is occluded, and autoregulation, which maintains constant blood flow through vasodilation or constriction.
2. When a patient has a seizure, the nurse should observe and record aura, incontinence, initial movement, respiratory pattern, duration of the seizure, loss of consciousness, and pupillary changes.
3. The major causes of cerebrovascular accident include thrombosis, embolism, and hemorrhage.
4. A positive response to Brudzinski's or Kernig's tests, or both, indicates meningeal inflammation, as in meningitis.

CHAPTER 6

1. Skeletal muscles may be classified by location, action, size, shape, point of attachment, number of divisions, or orientation of fibers.
2. Bone renewal continues throughout life, but slows down with age.
3. Medications for gouty arthritis include uricosuric agents, xanthine-oxidase inhibitors, antigout agents, analgesics, intra-articular corticosteroids, and nonsteroidal anti-inflammatory drugs.

4. Osteoporosis is characterized by porous and brittle bones that are abnormally vulnerable to fracture.

CHAPTER 7

1. Scarlet fever is a group A streptococcal infection.
2. *Salmonella* may be transmitted by contaminated dry milk, chocolate bars, or pharmaceuticals of animal origin or through contaminated or inadequately processed foods, especially eggs, chickens, turkeys, and ducks.
3. A bull's-eye–shaped rash is a distinctive early sign of Lyme disease. The rash is commonly accompanied by fatigue, malaise, headache, fever, sore throat, stiff neck, nausea, muscle and joint pain, and lymphadenopathy.
4. *Hantavirus* pulmonary syndrome was first reported in 1993. It is transmitted by contact with infected rodents or their wastes, and by ingestion of contaminated food or water.
5. The rubella rash appears and disappears more rapidly than the rubeola (measles) rash.

CHAPTER 8

1. Immunoglobulin E (IgE) is involved in the immediate hypersensitivity reactions of humoral immunity. Within minutes of exposure to an antigen, IgE stimulates the release of mast cell granules, which contain histamine, heparin, and other mediators.
2. Three common complaints in rheumatoid arthritis include painful joints, weak muscles, and peripheral neuropathy, which commonly develops in the fingers and extends bilaterally to the wrists, elbows, knees, and ankles.
3. About half of all lupus patients develop a characteristic butterfly rash over their noses and cheeks. Other common signs and symptoms include: fever, anorexia, weight loss, malaise, fatigue, abdominal pain, nausea, vomiting, diarrhea, constipation, rashes, polyarthralgia, and photosensitivity. About 90% of patients also have joint pain resembling rheumatoid arthritis.
4. HIV is transmitted by contact with infected blood or blood products and infected body fluids. It also crosses the placenta from the infected mother to the fetus, and passes in breast milk to the neonate.

CHAPTER 9

1. The patient with gastritis should avoid caffeine, alcohol, and spicy or fried foods.
2. Ulcerative colitis damages the large intestine's mucosal and submucosal layers.
3. Possible causes of Crohn's disease include lymphatic obstruction, infection, allergies, immune disorders, and genetic factors.
4. Although an obstruction may initiate some cases of appendicitis, ulceration of the mucosa is the usual initial event.

CHAPTER 10

1. Type A hepatitis virus is transmitted through oral ingestion of fecal-contaminated food and liquids as well as by sexual (especially oral-anal) contact. Type B hepatitis virus is transmitted by blood and body fluids.
2. Pyogenic liver abscess results from infection by *Escherichia coli, Klebsiella, Enterobacter, Salmonella, Staphylococcus, Enterococcus,* and *Streptococcus.*
3. The diet regimen for cirrhosis is high-calorie, high-carbohydrate, low-fat, low-sodium, low-protein foods, given in small, frequent feedings. Alcohol and fluid intake is restricted.
4. If a nonsurgical approach is not effective, cholelithiasis is treated surgically by open or laparoscopic cholecystectomy.

CHAPTER 11

1. The three key functions of the renal system are collecting and removing waste products from the blood, maintaining blood pressure, and regulating electrolyte concentration and acid-base balance of body fluids.
2. The most common cause of acute renal failure (75% of cases) is acute tubular necrosis.
3. Prerenal failure results from any condition that diminishes blood flow to the kidney.
4. Acute poststreptococcal glomerulonephritis usually follows a respiratory streptococcal infection, or, in some cases, a skin infection

such as impetigo, or infection with group A beta-hemolytic streptococcus.

5. Causes of metabolic acidosis include diabetic ketoacidosis, starvation, renal failure, poisoning, diarrhea, lactic acidosis, intestinal fistulas, and administration of large amounts of normal saline solution or ammonium chloride.

CHAPTER 12

1. Possible assessment findings for hypothyroidism include fatigue, weight gain, dry flaky skin, edema, intolerance to cold, coarse hair, thickened tongue, swollen lips, mental sluggishness, menstrual disorders, constipation, hypersensitivity to drugs, anorexia, decreased diaphoresis, and hypothermia.
2. Graves' disease, the most common hyperthyroid disorder, is an autoimmune disorder that causes goiter, exophthalmos, dermopathy, and multiple systemic changes.
3. Signs and symptoms of Addison's disease include weight loss, GI disturbances, dehydration, fatigue, muscle weakness, anxiety, light-headedness, amenorrhea, and craving for salty foods.
4. Cushing's syndrome may be caused by excessive glucocorticoids (hypercortisolism) or excess androgen secretion. The primary form is usually caused by an adrenal tumor; the secondary form (also called Cushing's disease) is usually caused by anterior pituitary hypofunction; the ter-

tiary form is usually caused by hypothalamic dysfunction or injury. Cushing's syndrome may also result from long-term therapy with exogenous corticosteroids.

5. Diabetes is classified as type 1, type 2 (most common), gestational, and other forms.

CHAPTER 13

1. *Escherichia coli* causes prostatitis in 80% of all cases.
2. In acute prostatitis, the prostate gland will feel abnormally hard, swollen, and warm.
3. In epididymitis, the waddling gait results from the patient's attempt to protect the painful groin and scrotum while walking.
4. A localized, hot, tender area in the testes might indicate possible abscess formation in epididymitis.
5. Signs and symptoms of possible urinary obstruction in benign prostatic hyperplasia include frequent urination with nocturia, dribbling, urine retention, incontinence, and hematuria.

CHAPTER 14

1. A patient with premenstrual syndrome should follow a diet low in simple sugars, caffeine, and salt.
2. In a patient with pelvic inflammatory disease, abdominal distention and rigidity are possible signs of developing peritonitis.

3. In endometriosis, pain usually begins 5 to 7 days before the menses.
4. Androgens, progestins, oral contraceptives, and gonadotropin-releasing hormone agonists are used to treat endometriosis.
5. Teach patients with fibrocystic breast changes to perform monthly self-breast examinations.

CHAPTER 15

1. The incubation period in chlamydia is 2 weeks.
2. Chlamydia is usually treated with doxycycline and azithromycin.
3. Condylomata acuminata is caused by the human papillomavirus.
4. Because certain types of human papillomavirus infections have been strongly linked to genital dysplasia and cervical neoplasia, annual Papanicolaou tests are recommended.
5. Patients with syphilis should have serologic tests done 3, 6, 12, and 24 months following treatment to monitor for relapse.

CHAPTER 16

1. Age-related macular degeneration occurs in a dry (atrophic) form and a wet (exudative) form.
2. Acute angle-closure glaucoma can cause blindness in 3 to 5 days.
3. After a myringotomy, position the patient on the affected side to facilitate drainage.

4. Four characteristic findings in Ménière's disease are severe rotary vertigo, tinnitus, sensorineural hearing loss, and a feeling of fullness in the ear.
5. Continuous mucopurulent nasal drainage results from chronic sinusitis.

CHAPTER 17

1. Atopic dermatitis is exacerbated by temperature and humidity extremes, emotional stress, allergens, and irritants such as wool or lanolin.
2. Psoriatic plaques develop characteristic silvery scales that either flake off easily or thicken.
3. Warts are caused by the human papillomavirus.
4. Warts can be transmitted by direct contact or, possibly, by autoinoculation.

CHAPTER 18

1. To feed an infant with cleft lip or palate, hold him in near-sitting position, with flow directed to the sides or back of the tongue. Also try using a nipple with a flange or a regular nipple with enlarged holes.
2. A patient with cystic fibrosis must take pancreatic enzymes with meals to prevent malabsorption and steatorrhea.
3. A patient with Down syndrome has 47 chromosomes because chromosome 21 forms 3 copies instead of the normal pair.

4. Untreated phenylketonuria will lead to cerebral damage with resulting mental retardation.
5. Sickle cell crisis is not evident until after age 6 months because the infant is protected by large amounts of fetal hemoglobin until he is this age.
6. Sickle cell crisis can be triggered by any condition that causes cellular hypoxia, such as infection, overexertion, or exposure to cold or high altitudes.

CHAPTER 19

1. Signs and symptoms of intracranial pressure include headache, vomiting, pupillary dysfunction, motor dysfunction, papilledema, and visual changes.
2. Adenocarcinoma of the breast is the most common form of breast cancer.
3. A high-fat, low-fiber diet may contribute to colorectal cancer by slowing fecal movement through the bowel.
4. Teach the patient with skin cancer to avoid overexposure to the sun and to use a strong sunscreen when outdoors.
5. A change in the shape, color and texture of a nevus may indicate malignant melanoma.

Selected References

Black, J.M., and Matassarin-Jacobs, E., eds. *Medical-Surgical Nursing: Clinical Management for Continuity of Care,* 5th ed. Philadelphia: W.B. Saunders Co., 1997.

Fanning, M.M. *HIV Infection: A Clinical Approach,* 2nd ed. Philadelphia: W.B. Saunders Co., 1997.

Hickey, J.V. *The Clinical Practice of Neurological and Neurosurgical Nursing,* 4th ed. Lippincott-Raven Pubs., 1997.

Kelley, W.N., et al., eds. *Textbook of Internal Medicine,* 3rd ed. Philadelphia: Lippincott-Raven Pubs., 1997.

Lemone, P. *Medical-Surgical Nursing: Critical Thinking in Client Care.* Reading, Mass.: Addison-Wesley-Longman Publishing Co., 1996.

McPhee, S.J., et al. *Pathophysiology of Disease: An Introduction to Clinical Medicine,* 2nd ed. Stamford, Conn.: Appleton & Lange, 1997.

Miaskowski, C. *Oncology Nursing: An Essential Guide for Patient Care.* Philadelphia: W.B. Saunders Co., 1997.

Pathophysiology Made Incredibly Easy. Springhouse, Pa.: Springhouse Corp. 1998.

Petty, T.L. *The 1997 Yearbook of Pulmonary Disease.* St. Louis: Mosby–Year Book, Inc., 1997.

Professional Guide to Diseases, 6th ed. Springhouse, Pa.: Springhouse Corp., 1997.

Smeltzer, S.C., and Bare, B.G. *Brunner and Suddarth's Textbook of Medical-Surgical Nursing,* 8th ed. Philadelphia: Lippincott-Raven Pubs., 1996.

Wright, K. *Textbook of Ophthalmology.* Baltimore: Williams & Wilkins Co., 1997.

Index

t refers to a table.

t refers to a table.

Notes

Notes

Notes

Notes

Notes

About the
StudySmart Disk

StudySmart Disk lets you:

- review subject areas of your choice and learn the rationales for the correct answers
- take tests of varying lengths on subjects of your choice
- print the results of your tests to gauge your progress over time.

Recommended system requirements
486 IBM-compatible personal computer
Windows 3.1 or greater (Windows® 95 compatible)
High-density 3½" floppy drive
16 MB RAM (8 MB minimum)
S-VGA monitor (VGA minimum)
2 MB of available space on hard drive

Installing and running the program
- Start Windows® 95.
- Select Start button and then Run.
- Insert disk, type a:\setup.exe (where a: is the letter of your floppy drive), and click OK.

For Windows 3.1 Installation
- Start Windows.
- In Program Manager, choose Run from File menu.
- Insert disk, type a:\setup.exe (where a: is the letter of your floppy drive), and click OK.

For technical support, call 1-877-872-7748 Monday through Friday, 8 a.m. to 5 p.m. Eastern Standard Time.

The clinical information and tools in the StudySmart Disk are based on research and consultation with nursing, medical, and legal authorities. To the best of our knowledge, the program reflects currently accepted practice; nevertheless, it can't be considered absolute or universal. For individual application, all recommendations must be considered in light of the patient's clinical condition and, before administration of new or infrequently used drugs, in light of the latest package-insert information. The authors and publisher disclaim responsibility for any adverse effects resulting directly or indirectly from the suggested procedures, from any undetected errors, or from the reader's misunderstanding of the program.